The Fourth Trimester

The Simplest Baby Guide For a Healthy Baby and The New Mom

Lindy

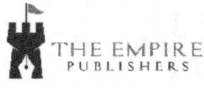

12808 West Airport Blvd Suite 270M Sugar Land, TX 77478, Unites States

https://www.theempirepublishers.com/

Our books may be purchased in bulk for promotional, educational, or business use.

Please contact The Empire Publishers at +1 844 636-4579, or by email at support@theempirepublishers.com

First Edition February 2025

To my incredible family,

Your unwavering love and support are the foundation of all that I do.

To my two amazing daughters, thank you for the boundless joy you've brought into my life and for blessing me with six beautiful grandchildren. Watching you both grow into wonderful mothers has been one of my greatest honors, and seeing my grandchildren thrive fills my heart with immeasurable pride.

To my husband and children, your love is my inspiration, and your encouragement fuels my passion for helping others. This work is a reflection of all the lessons we've shared and the strength we've built together as a family.

With love and gratitude,

Lindy

About the Author

Lindy is a devoted wife and mother to five children, a role she cherishes deeply. She holds a doctorate (PhD) in Naturopathic Medicine, a field she is passionate about and has dedicated her life to. With a strong belief in the power of natural remedies, Lindy advocates for the use of herbs as an essential aid in promoting health and well-being through naturopathic principles.

Over the years, Lindy has been a guiding light for countless new mothers, offering support and advice to help them navigate the physical and emotional challenges that often accompany childbirth. Through her expertise and compassionate approach, she has provided practical solutions for managing postpartum recovery and has empowered women to embrace holistic health practices.

Lindy has also shared her knowledge by hosting classes designed to help new moms prioritize self-care while balancing the demands of family life. Her emphasis on mental health as a cornerstone of effective motherhood has resonated with many, inspiring women to take care of themselves so they can nurture their families more effectively.

In addition to her professional work, Lindy is an avid learner and educator who is continually seeking new ways to enhance the lives of those she works with. Her dedication to promoting holistic wellness and supporting mothers in their journeys makes her a trusted voice in the field of naturopathic medicine.

Table of Contents

Introduction

Bringing my first baby home was a whirlwind of emotions. I remember feeling a mix of overwhelming joy and sheer exhaustion. There were moments when I looked at my newborn daughter and felt an immense love I had never known was possible. But there were also times when I felt utterly lost and unsure if I was doing anything right. During these early weeks—often referred to as the fourth trimester—I realized how crucial this period is for both the baby and the new mother.

The fourth trimester refers to the first three months after childbirth. It is a time of profound change and adaptation. For the baby, it involves adjusting to life outside the womb. For the new mother, it is a period of physical recovery and emotional transition. Understanding and navigating this time can make a huge difference in ensuring a healthy start for both.

The primary goal of this book is to provide simple, practical guidance for new mothers. My aim is to help you ensure a healthy baby and a healthy postpartum period for yourself. This book focuses on key areas like sleep training, feeding, and self-care—building blocks for a smoother transition into motherhood.

This guide is designed for new mothers, especially first-time moms. If you are navigating the unknowns of the postpartum period, you are in the right place. Every new mother faces challenges, and this book aims to be your companion, offering support and advice when you need it most.

What sets this book apart from other baby guides is its integration of professional insights. I have included advice from pediatricians, nurses, lactation specialists, and a community of experienced mothers and fathers. This blend of expertise ensures that you get well-rounded, reliable information.

Allow me to introduce myself. I am Lindy Summers, a mother of five and a naturopathic doctor. I have dedicated my career to helping new mothers. My experience with postpartum care, including the use of herbs and leading classes for new moms, has given me a unique perspective. I understand the physical and emotional challenges you face, and I am here to help you navigate them.

This book is divided into several sections, each focusing on different aspects of the fourth trimester. You will find chapters on sleep training, feeding schedules, and newborn care. There are also sections on traveling with a baby, preparing the nursery, and managing common ailments. Each chapter offers practical tips and best practices.

New mothers often face common challenges during the fourth trimester. Sleep deprivation, feeding issues, and postpartum mental health struggles are frequent hurdles. This book provides practical solutions to these problems. You will find strategies to help you cope with sleep deprivation, tips for establishing effective feeding routines, and sections dedicated to mental health support.

I encourage you to actively use this book as a resource. Take notes, highlight important sections, and revisit chapters as needed. This book is meant to be a companion on your journey through the fourth trimester.

By the end of this book, I hope you will feel more confident and prepared to handle the fourth trimester. My goal is to foster a healthy, happy environment for both you and your baby. You are not alone in this journey. With the right guidance and support, you can navigate the fourth trimester successfully.

Remember, every new mother faces challenges. It is okay to ask for help and seek advice. You are doing an amazing job. With each passing day, you are becoming more confident and capable. Together, we can make the fourth trimester a positive, nurturing experience for you and your baby.

Chapter 1:
Navigating Mental Health

One afternoon, while rocking my newborn son to sleep, the weight of exhaustion and uncertainty hit me like a wave. I remember wondering if I was the only one feeling so overwhelmed. These emotions were a stark contrast to the joy I had expected to fill those early weeks. It was then that I realized the fourth trimester is not just about caring for your new baby but also about caring for yourself. This chapter is dedicated to helping you navigate the mental health challenges that often accompany this period.

Recognizing Postpartum Depression vs. Baby Blues

The first step in managing your mental health during the fourth trimester is understanding the difference between the baby blues and postpartum depression. Both conditions affect many new mothers, but they vary in severity and duration.

The baby blues are quite common and typically appear a few days after childbirth, lasting for about two weeks. You might experience mood swings, crying spells, and anxiety. These symptoms, while distressing, usually resolve on their own as your hormones stabilize.

Postpartum depression, on the other hand, is more intense and long-lasting. It can start within the first few weeks after delivery and may continue for several months or even longer. Symptoms include intense sadness, severe mood swings, and withdrawal from social activities. Unlike the baby blues, postpartum depression often requires professional treatment.

You might struggle to bond with your baby, feel hopeless, or even have thoughts of self-harm. Recognizing these symptoms early can lead to more effective treatment and quicker recovery.

It's important to know that you are not alone. According to the Mayo Clinic, postpartum depression affects around 12.7% of women who have recently given birth. Rates vary by location, with states like Vermont reporting lower rates (around 8.7%) and states like Idaho seeing rates as high as 25.4%. These statistics highlight the prevalence of postpartum depression and underscore the importance of seeking help if needed.

Personal stories can also be incredibly reassuring. Take Emily, a new mother from Georgia, who found herself crying uncontrollably at odd times. She felt guilty for not being constantly joyful around her newborn and worried she was failing as a mother. After talking to her healthcare provider, she realized she was experiencing postpartum depression. With a treatment plan that included therapy and medication, Emily gradually regained her confidence. Her story is a reminder that seeking help is a sign of strength, not weakness.

To help you gauge your mental health, here is a simple self-assessment checklist:

Self-Assessment Checklist

- Do you find yourself crying more often than usual?
- Are you experiencing severe mood swings that interfere with daily life?
- Do you feel an overwhelming sense of sadness or hopelessness?
- Are you having trouble bonding with your baby?
- Do you feel disconnected from family and friends?
- Are you sleeping too much or too little?

- Have you lost interest in activities you once enjoyed?
- Are you experiencing overwhelming fatigue that makes it hard to get through the day?
- Do you have thoughts of self-harm or harming your baby?

If you answered "yes" to several of these questions, it might be time to seek professional help. Early detection is crucial, as recognizing symptoms early can lead to more effective treatment and quicker recovery. The benefits of early intervention include improved mental health, better bonding with your baby, and a quicker return to your normal activities. On the other hand, untreated postpartum depression can lead to long-term consequences—not just for you, but for your child as well. It can affect your baby's cognitive and emotional development and strain your relationships with loved ones.

Understanding these conditions and knowing when to seek help can make a significant difference in your postpartum experience. You are not alone, and there are resources and support systems available to help you through this challenging time.

Practical Tips for Managing Postpartum Anxiety

Managing postpartum anxiety can be challenging, but there are actionable strategies you can use to find relief during those intense moments. One effective method is grounding techniques, which help you focus on the present moment by using your senses. For instance, when you feel anxiety creeping in, try to identify five things you can see, four things you can touch, three things you can hear, two things you can smell, and one thing you can taste. This simple exercise can help redirect your mind away from anxiety and toward your immediate surroundings. Another quick method is engaging in a short activity that you enjoy, such as listening to your favorite music or taking a few moments to read a chapter of a book. These distractions can offer a mental break and provide temporary relief from anxious thoughts.

In addition to these immediate strategies, incorporating regular mental health practices can make a significant difference in managing postpartum anxiety over time. Journaling is a powerful tool that allows you to reflect on your daily experiences and write down your worries. By putting your thoughts on paper, you can gain a clearer perspective and identify patterns that may be contributing to your anxiety. Make it a habit to set aside a few minutes each day to jot down your thoughts and feelings. Another helpful practice is building a daily routine that includes relaxation time. Establishing a consistent schedule can provide a sense of stability and predictability, which can be calming. Incorporate activities that bring you joy and relaxation, such as a warm bath, reading a book, or spending time outdoors.

Physical activity also plays a crucial role in managing anxiety. Gentle exercises, like postpartum yoga, can help alleviate anxiety symptoms by promoting relaxation and improving overall well-being. Specific yoga poses, such as child's pose and cat-cow stretch, are particularly effective for reducing stress and tension. These poses can be easily done at home and require minimal equipment. Walking is another excellent form of exercise that offers multiple benefits. The combination of fresh air, light physical activity, and a change of scenery can work wonders for your mental state. Aim for a daily walk, even if it's just a short stroll around the neighborhood. The rhythmic motion of walking can have a soothing effect and give you a much-needed mental break.

Diet and sleep are fundamental aspects of managing anxiety. Maintaining a balanced diet can significantly impact your mood and energy levels. Incorporate foods that boost mood, such as fruits, vegetables, lean proteins, and whole grains. Staying hydrated is equally important, so make sure to drink plenty of water throughout the day. Avoid excessive caffeine and sugar, as they can contribute to anxiety and mood swings. Sleep hygiene is another critical factor. Creating a sleep-friendly environment can improve the quality of your rest, which in turn helps manage anxiety. Keep your bedroom cool, dark, and quiet. Establish a bedtime routine that signals to your body that it's time to wind down. This might include activities like reading a book, listening to calming music, or practicing deep breathing exercises.

When anxiety strikes, it can feel overwhelming, but these practical tips offer various ways to manage and alleviate those feelings. By focusing on immediate relief through grounding techniques and distractions and incorporating regular mental health practices, physical activity, a balanced diet, and good sleep hygiene, you can create a comprehensive approach to managing postpartum anxiety. Remember, it's essential to take care of yourself—not just for your well-being but also for your ability to care for your baby.

1.3 Mindfulness Exercises for New Moms

Mindfulness is a practice that involves paying full attention to the present moment without judgment. It's about being aware of your thoughts, feelings, and sensations as they occur. For new mothers, mindfulness can be a powerful tool to reduce stress and improve focus. Instead of getting lost in worries about the future or regrets about the past, mindfulness helps you stay grounded in the here and now. This can be particularly beneficial during the fourth trimester when life is filled with new challenges and adjustments.

One of the simplest yet most effective mindfulness exercises is mindful breathing. This practice involves focusing on your breath, noticing each inhale and exhale without trying to change it. Find a quiet spot where you won't be disturbed. Sit comfortably, close your eyes, and take a deep breath in through your nose, counting to four. Hold the breath for a count of four, then exhale slowly through your mouth for a count of six. Repeat this process for a few minutes, allowing your mind to settle and your body to relax. This exercise can be done anytime, whether you're feeling overwhelmed or just need a moment of calm.

Another beneficial mindfulness practice is the body scan meditation. This exercise helps you pay attention to different parts of your body, releasing any tension you might be holding. Start by lying down in a comfortable position. Close your eyes and take a few deep breaths. Begin by focusing on your toes, noticing any sensations, and then gradually move your attention up through your legs, torso, arms, and head. As you focus on each body part, consciously release any tension you find. This exercise can be particularly helpful before bed, as it promotes relaxation and can improve sleep quality.

Mindfulness can also be incorporated into daily routines, turning everyday tasks into moments of calm and presence. For example, mindful eating involves savoring each bite of food, paying attention to the flavors, textures, and sensations. Instead of rushing through meals, take time to enjoy them. This not only enhances your eating experience but also promotes better digestion and helps you recognize when you're full. Another practical application is mindful baby care. When you're changing a diaper or feeding your baby, focus entirely on the task at hand. Notice your baby's expressions, the feel of their skin, and the sounds they make. Being fully present during these moments can strengthen your bond with your baby and make routine tasks more enjoyable.

Consistency and patience are key to mindfulness. It's important to set realistic goals for your practice. Start with short sessions—just a few minutes each day—and gradually increase the time as you become more comfortable. Remember, mindfulness is a skill that takes time to develop. Some days will feel easier than others, and that's perfectly normal. Be kind to yourself and accept fluctuations in your practice as part of the journey.

Incorporating mindfulness into daily life can bring calm and clarity to the often chaotic fourth trimester. By focusing on the present moment, you can reduce stress, improve your mood, and enhance your overall well-being. Whether through mindful breathing, body scan meditations, or simply being present during everyday tasks, mindfulness offers a range of benefits to help you navigate the early months of motherhood with greater ease.

1.4 Breathing Techniques to Alleviate Stress

Understanding the science behind breathing techniques highlights why they are so effective for stress relief. When you control your breathing, you activate the parasympathetic nervous system, which promotes relaxation and counteracts the body's fight-or-flight response. Engaging this system lowers your heart rate and reduces levels of stress hormones like cortisol, creating an almost immediate calming effect. These techniques are simple and can be practiced anywhere.

One effective exercise is diaphragmatic breathing, or "belly breathing." Sit or lie comfortably, placing one hand on your chest and the other on your belly. Inhale deeply through your nose, allowing your diaphragm to expand and push your belly upward. Your chest should remain relatively still. Exhale slowly through your mouth, feeling your belly fall. Repeat several times, focusing on the gentle rise and fall of your belly. This method promotes deeper, more efficient breathing and calms the mind.

Another technique is box breathing, which involves equal counts for inhaling, holding, exhaling, and holding again. Sit comfortably, close your eyes if you wish, and inhale through your nose for four counts. Hold your breath for four counts, exhale through your mouth for four counts, and hold again for four counts. Repeat this cycle several times to regulate your breathing and foster a sense of control, especially during stressful moments.

The 4-7-8 breathing technique is also powerful. Sit or lie comfortably, inhale quietly through your nose for four counts, hold your breath for seven counts, then exhale completely through your mouth for eight counts. Repeat three to four times. This technique is particularly effective at bedtime, helping calm your mind and prepare your body for restful sleep.

Integrating these exercises into your daily routine offers ongoing stress relief. Diaphragmatic breathing before sleep can help you transition from the day's busyness to relaxation, improving sleep quality. During feeding times, use box breathing to center yourself, allowing its rhythm to soothe both you and your baby. In moments of sudden stress, such as when your baby is inconsolable, a quick session of 4-7-8 breathing can reset your mental state and provide immediate relief.

The effectiveness of these exercises cannot be overstated. One mother shared how diaphragmatic breathing helped her regain calm during late-night feedings, turning anxiety into manageable moments. Another mother found box breathing invaluable during her baby's colic episodes, staying grounded and responding with greater patience.

My own experience with 4-7-8 breathing has been transformative. I recall a particularly challenging day when my baby was fussy, and I felt utterly drained. After just a few minutes of 4-7-8 breathing, my heart rate slowed, my mind cleared, and I felt a newfound sense of control. These techniques aren't just stress-management tools; they are lifelines for reclaiming peace and stability amid chaos.

1.5 Building a Support Network for Mental Health

Having a strong support network during the fourth trimester is crucial for mental health. Emotional support can make a significant difference, especially when you feel overwhelmed or anxious. Feeling understood and validated by those around you provides comfort and reassurance, making new motherhood's challenges more manageable. Practical support is equally important. Assistance with daily tasks—like cooking, cleaning, and childcare—frees up time and energy, allowing you to focus on bonding with your baby and caring for yourself. Together, emotional and practical support create a more balanced and less stressful environment for you and your baby.

Building a support network begins with reaching out to family and friends. Don't hesitate to ask for specific help. While it might feel uncomfortable at first, most people are eager to lend a hand. Whether it's requesting a friend to bring over a meal or asking a family member to watch the baby for a few hours, clear requests make it easier for others to support you effectively. Additionally, local parenting groups can be a valuable resource.

These groups offer a sense of community and shared experiences. You can find them through community centers, hospitals, or social media. Joining a local parenting group can provide firsthand advice, emotional support, and a sense of belonging.

Online communities can also be a lifeline for new mothers. Virtual spaces like forums, social media groups, and specialized apps offer support from others who understand what you're going through. These platforms allow you to connect anytime, providing immediate advice and reassurance. Sharing experiences, asking questions, and receiving feedback from diverse parents can be especially valuable during late-night feedings when you might feel isolated.

Professional support options should not be overlooked. Postpartum doulas can provide tailored emotional and practical support. Trained to help new mothers adjust to life with a newborn, they offer guidance on breastfeeding, infant care, and self-care. Recommendations can be obtained from healthcare providers or online directories. Therapists specializing in postpartum care can also help by providing coping strategies and emotional support. Look for professionals experienced in maternal mental health, and consider referrals from your healthcare provider.

Open communication is essential for maintaining a strong support network. Clearly expressing your needs and feelings using "I" statements can avoid sounding accusatory. For example, saying, "I feel overwhelmed and could use help with the baby" is more effective than "You never help me with the baby." Clear communication helps others understand how they can better support you. Additionally, setting boundaries is crucial—know when to say no to extra responsibilities or social engagements that might increase your stress. Prioritizing your mental health is okay.

Building and maintaining a support network requires effort, but the benefits are worth it. Emotional and practical support can significantly enhance your mental health, providing the strength and resilience needed to face the challenges of the fourth trimester. Whether from family, friends, local parenting groups, online communities, or professionals, a strong support system makes this period more manageable and less isolating. Remember, asking for help and leaning on others during this time is okay—you don't have to do it all alone.

When to Seek Professional Help

Knowing when to seek professional help is crucial for your well-being and your baby's. Persistent sadness lasting more than two weeks is a clear indicator that it's time to consult a professional. Other critical signs include thoughts of self-harm or harming your baby—these require immediate attention. Severe anxiety that interferes with daily functioning is another red flag. If completing everyday tasks feels impossible or if anxiety prevents you from enjoying time with your baby, seeking professional help is essential.

Various professionals can assist with postpartum mental health. Psychologists offer therapy that helps you navigate emotions and develop coping strategies. Psychiatrists can manage medication when therapy alone is insufficient, providing significant symptom relief. Support groups— whether in person or online—offer peer-led discussions for comfort and practical advice. Connecting with other mothers facing similar challenges fosters a sense of community and understanding.

Finding the right professional may seem daunting, but there are steps to ensure the best care. Start by verifying credentials to confirm expertise in postpartum care. Many therapists and psychiatrists specialize in maternal mental health, enhancing the quality of care. Seek recommendations from trusted sources like healthcare providers or friends who've had similar experiences. Don't hesitate to ask potential professionals about their experience and treatment approach.

The benefits of professional intervention are profound. Many mothers report significant improvements in mental health after seeking help. For example, Sarah, a mother from California, overcame severe postpartum depression through therapy and medication. She noticed dramatic improvements in her mood and energy, feeling more connected to her baby and capable of managing daily tasks. Another mother, Jessica, found relief by joining a support group. Sharing experiences with peers made her feel less isolated and more understood.

Professional help also benefits your relationship with your baby. Improved mental health enhances bonding and the overall parenting experience, fostering confidence and capability. Addressing mental health issues early can prevent them from escalating, improving relationships with your partner and family.

In conclusion, recognizing when to seek professional help is a vital step for a healthy postpartum period. Persistent sadness, self-harm thoughts, and severe anxiety indicate the need for intervention. Psychologists, psychiatrists, and support groups offer valuable assistance. By verifying credentials and seeking recommendations, you can find the right professional. The benefits of intervention are significant, improving mental health and parenting experiences. Seeking help demonstrates strength and ensures the best care for yourself and your baby.

Chapter 2:
Physical Recovery and Well-Being

I remember the first time I stood up after my C-section. My legs felt wobbly, and the incision site throbbed with every movement. Holding my newborn son in my arms, I realized that my body had undergone major surgery and that recovery would take time and patience. This chapter focuses on your physical recovery and well-being, offering practical advice and insights to help you heal and regain your strength.

Healing After a C-Section
The recovery process after a C-section involves several stages, each with its own challenges and milestones. Immediately after the surgery, you will likely feel groggy from the anesthesia and may experience pain at the incision site. In the hospital, you will receive IV fluids and a light meal within 6–8 hours post-surgery. Pain management is crucial during this period, with long-acting medications and Toradol to help alleviate discomfort. You may also experience postpartum cramping, constipation, and gas pains. It's important to begin breastfeeding and walking as soon as possible, as these activities promote healing and help prevent complications like blood clots.

During the first few weeks after a C-section, your focus should be on gradually increasing physical activity while managing pain and monitoring the incision site. Pain may persist but should gradually decrease over time. Oral pain medications, such as acetaminophen or ibuprofen, can help manage discomfort. Non-pharmacological methods, like heat packs and gentle massage, can also provide relief. It's important to remove the bandage and Foley catheter within the first day, and your healthcare provider will monitor your progress and remove any sutures or staples as needed.

As you enter the long-term healing phase, scar care becomes a priority. Keeping the incision clean and dry is essential to prevent infection and promote healing. Use mild soap and water to gently clean the area, and pat it dry with a clean towel. Avoid submerging the incision in water, such as during baths or swimming, until your healthcare provider gives you the go-ahead. Watch for signs of infection, including redness, swelling, and fever. If you notice any of these symptoms, contact your healthcare provider immediately. Over time, the scar will fade, but you may experience lingering discomfort or numbness around the incision site. Gentle massage and silicone gel sheets can help improve the appearance of the scar and reduce discomfort.

Rest and limited activity are crucial during the recovery process. Your body needs time to heal, and overexertion can lead to complications. Prioritize rest and avoid heavy lifting or strenuous tasks. Gradually increase your activity level by incorporating light exercise, such as walking, into your daily routine. Walking promotes circulation and helps prevent blood clots, but be sure to listen to your body and avoid pushing yourself too hard. Most healthcare providers recommend waiting 6–8 weeks before resuming moderate exercise, such as yoga or Pilates.

In those early weeks, it's important to manage pain and

discomfort effectively. Pain medication can be a valuable tool, but it's essential to use it safely. Follow your healthcare provider's instructions and avoid taking more than the recommended dose. Non-pharmacological pain relief methods, such as heat packs and gentle massage, can complement medication and provide additional comfort. Heat packs can help relax tense muscles and reduce pain, while gentle massage can promote circulation and alleviate discomfort around the incision site.

Caring for your incision is a critical aspect of the recovery process. Keep the incision clean and dry to prevent infection and promote healing. Use mild soap and water to gently clean the area, and pat it dry with a clean towel. Avoid using harsh chemicals or scrubbing the incision, as this can irritate the skin and delay healing. Watch for signs of infection, such as redness, swelling, and fever. If you notice any of these symptoms, contact your healthcare provider immediately. Keeping the area dry is also important, so avoid submerging the incision in water until your healthcare provider gives you the green light.

C-Section Recovery Checklist
- **Keep the incision clean and dry**: Use mild soap and water, and avoid submerging in water.
- **Monitor for signs of infection**: Watch for redness, swelling, and fever.
- **Manage pain effectively**: Use prescribed pain medications and non-pharmacological methods.
- **Prioritize rest**: Avoid heavy lifting and strenuous tasks.
- **Gradually increase activity**: Incorporate light exercise, such as walking, into your daily routine.
- **Scar care**: Use gentle massage and silicone gel sheets to improve appearance and reduce discomfort.

Managing your physical recovery after a C-section requires patience and self-care. By following these guidelines and listening to your body, you can promote healing and regain your strength. Remember, every mother's recovery journey is unique, and it's important to be kind to yourself during this time.

Pelvic Floor Strengthening Exercises
Pelvic floor health is often overlooked but is incredibly important after childbirth. Strengthening your pelvic floor muscles can significantly improve bladder control and reduce discomfort. Neglecting these muscles can lead to issues such as incontinence and pelvic organ prolapse. The pelvic floor supports the uterus, bladder, and bowel. During pregnancy and childbirth, these muscles can become weakened, resulting in a range of issues that can affect your quality of life. Taking steps to strengthen them can enhance your recovery and overall well-being.

Kegel exercises are one of the most effective ways to strengthen the pelvic floor. First, you need to identify the right muscles. An easy way to do this is by trying to stop your urine midstream. The muscles you use to do this are your pelvic floor muscles. Once you have identified them, you can begin practicing Kegel exercises. Sit comfortably and contract these muscles for three to five seconds, then relax for the same amount of time. It's important to avoid using your abdominal, thigh, or buttock muscles. Aim to do at least three sets of ten repetitions each day. Consistency is key, and with regular practice, you should start to see improvements within a few weeks to a few months.

In addition to Kegel exercises, other movements can help strengthen your pelvic floor. The bridge pose is an excellent exercise that targets these muscles. Lie on your back with your knees bent and feet flat on the floor. Slowly lift your hips towards the ceiling, squeezing your pelvic floor muscles as you rise. Hold the position for a few seconds before lowering your hips back down. Another effective exercise is squats. Stand with your feet shoulder-width apart and lower your body as if you're sitting in a chair, ensuring your knees do not extend past your toes. Squats not only strengthen the pelvic floor but also work the glutes and thighs. Performing these exercises correctly and regularly can improve muscle tone and function. Sometimes, professional help may be necessary for pelvic floor issues. If you experience persistent pain, incontinence that doesn't improve, or symptoms like a feeling of heaviness in the pelvic area, it's time to consult a specialist. A pelvic floor specialist can provide tailored exercises and treatments to address your specific needs. Referrals from your healthcare provider can help you find the right professional. Expect a thorough evaluation, including a physical examination, to determine the best course of action for your recovery.

Reflection Section: Is it Time to Consult a Specialist?
- Are you experiencing ongoing pain that doesn't improve with Kegel exercises?
- Do you have persistent urinary incontinence or difficulty controlling bowel movements?
- Have you noticed a feeling of heaviness or bulging in the pelvic area?
- Are these issues affecting your daily life and well-being?

If you answered "yes" to any of these questions, it might be time to seek professional help. Your healthcare provider can refer you to a pelvic floor specialist who can offer targeted treatments and support. Don't hesitate to reach out for help—improving your pelvic floor health can significantly enhance your quality of life.

Taking care of your pelvic floor is an important aspect of postpartum recovery. By incorporating Kegel exercises and other pelvic floor movements into your daily routine, you can improve muscle strength and function. If you experience persistent issues, consulting a specialist can provide the additional support you need. Strengthening your pelvic floor not only aids recovery but also enhances your overall well-being.

Nutritional Tips for Postpartum Recovery

Nutrition plays a pivotal role in your postpartum recovery, influencing everything from tissue repair to energy levels. After childbirth, your body needs to heal, and the right nutrients can make a significant difference. A balanced diet rich in essential vitamins and minerals supports the repair of tissues that were stretched or torn during delivery. Nutrients like vitamin C and zinc are particularly beneficial for skin health and tissue repair. Consuming foods high in these nutrients can help accelerate healing, allowing you to feel better faster.

Additionally, maintaining your energy levels is crucial. Breastfeeding, sleepless nights, and the demands of caring for a newborn can be exhausting. Proper nutrition ensures you have the stamina to meet these challenges head-on.

Key nutrients needed for postpartum recovery include protein, iron, calcium, and omega-3 fatty acids. Protein is vital for muscle repair and overall recovery. Lean meats, dairy products, and legumes are excellent sources of protein. Incorporating these into your meals can help you regain strength and support your body's healing process. Iron is another crucial nutrient, especially if you experienced significant blood loss during delivery. Leafy greens, red meat, and fortified cereals can help replenish your iron levels, reducing the risk of anemia and boosting your energy.

Calcium is essential for bone health, particularly if you are breastfeeding. Dairy products and fortified plant-based milks are good sources of calcium. Omega-3 fatty acids are beneficial for both you and your baby, supporting brain health and reducing inflammation. Fish like salmon and flaxseeds are rich in omega-3s.

Planning nutritious meals can seem overwhelming, especially when you're caring for a newborn. However, simple, quick meal ideas can make a big difference. Smoothies packed with fruits, vegetables, and a scoop of protein powder are easy to prepare and nutrient-dense. Salads with a variety of colorful vegetables, lean protein, and a healthy fat source like avocado can be both satisfying and nourishing. One-pot dishes such as stir-fries or casseroles can save time and reduce cleanup. For snacks, consider options like nuts, yogurt, and fruit—easy to grab and packed with essential nutrients to keep your energy stable throughout the day.

Hydration is another critical aspect of postpartum recovery. Adequate fluid intake is essential for tissue repair, energy levels, and breastfeeding. Aim to drink at least eight glasses of water a day. Hydrating beverages like herbal teas can also be beneficial, offering both hydration and additional nutrients. Chamomile tea, for example, can be soothing and promote relaxation, while peppermint tea can aid digestion. Keep a water bottle within reach throughout the day to remind yourself to stay hydrated. Dehydration can lead to fatigue and make recovery more challenging, so make hydration a priority.

Quick Meal Ideas and Snacks
- **Smoothies:** Blend spinach, banana, Greek yogurt, and a handful of berries for a quick, nutrient-packed breakfast.
- **Salads:** Toss together mixed greens, grilled chicken,

cherry tomatoes, and avocado, drizzling with olive oil and lemon juice.

- **One-Pot Dishes:** Prepare a chicken and vegetable stir-fry with brown rice in one pan for an easy dinner.
- **Snacks:** Keep a bowl of mixed nuts and dried fruit on hand, or enjoy a cup of Greek yogurt topped with honey and fresh berries.

Incorporating these nutritional tips into your daily routine can significantly aid postpartum recovery. A balanced diet rich in essential nutrients supports tissue repair, maintains energy levels, and enhances overall well-being. Quick meal ideas and healthy snacks can make it easier to stay nourished even when time is limited. And remember, hydration is key—keep those fluids flowing to support your body as it heals and adjusts to the demands of motherhood.

Managing Postpartum Pain

Postpartum pain manifests in various ways and can feel overwhelming. Perineal pain is common after a vaginal delivery, especially if tearing or an episiotomy occurred. This discomfort can make everyday activities like sitting or walking difficult. Uterine contractions, also known as afterpains, are another source of discomfort. These contractions help the uterus return to its pre-pregnancy size but can be painful, particularly during breastfeeding. Breast discomfort, such as engorgement or nipple pain, is also frequent and can make breastfeeding a challenging experience.

Effectively managing these types of pain can significantly improve your postpartum recovery. Over-the-counter pain relievers like ibuprofen or acetaminophen can help with perineal and uterine pain. These medications are generally safe while breastfeeding, but always consult your healthcare provider before use. Non-pharmacological methods are also beneficial. For example, sitz baths, where you soak the perineal area in warm water for 15–20 minutes, can reduce swelling and promote healing. Cold packs are another effective option for reducing inflammation and numbing the area.

Physical therapy can play a key role in managing postpartum pain. A physical therapist can create a personalized plan with targeted exercises to strengthen your core and pelvic floor muscles. These exercises not only alleviate pain but also improve overall physical function. Seeking professional guidance ensures exercises are performed correctly, maximizing their benefits while minimizing injury risks. Your healthcare provider can refer you to a qualified therapist specializing in postpartum care. Typically, therapy begins with an assessment followed by a tailored exercise program.

Communicating your pain to healthcare providers is crucial for receiving appropriate treatment. Keeping a pain diary can be especially helpful. Record your symptoms, noting when pain occurs, its intensity, and any factors that worsen or relieve it. Use specific terms like "sharp," "dull," "throbbing," or "constant" to describe your discomfort. A pain scale (e.g., rating pain from 1 to 10) can also give your provider a clearer picture of your condition. This clear communication enables your provider to create an effective treatment plan.

For perineal pain, particularly from tearing or an episiotomy, over-the-counter pain relievers can provide relief. Sitz baths are a soothing alternative; sitting in warm water for 15–20 minutes several times a day can reduce swelling and aid healing. Cold packs can numb the area and ease inflammation. If discomfort persists, consult your healthcare provider for additional options.

Uterine contractions, or afterpains, are another common

postpartum challenge. These contractions, often more pronounced during breastfeeding due to oxytocin release, aid the healing process. Over-the-counter pain relievers like acetaminophen can help, as can relaxation techniques such as deep breathing or gentle abdominal massages. While afterpains can be uncomfortable, they signal your body is healing.

Breast discomfort, whether from engorgement or nipple pain, is also typical. Engorgement, caused by overly full breasts, can make them feel hard and painful. Frequent breastfeeding or pumping can alleviate this discomfort. Warm compresses before feeding and cold packs afterward can provide additional relief. Nipple pain, often due to improper latching, can be addressed by consulting a lactation specialist. They can guide you on achieving a proper latch and recommend soothing nipple creams.

Physical therapy offers long-term benefits for postpartum pain management. A specialist can guide you through targeted exercises that strengthen weakened muscles and strained ligaments. These exercises promote pain relief and overall recovery. Finding a qualified therapist through referrals from your healthcare provider ensures you receive tailored care for your needs.

Managing postpartum pain involves a combination of strategies. From over-the-counter medications to non-pharmacological methods like sitz baths and cold packs, and professional physical therapy, relief is achievable. Clear communication with your healthcare provider about your pain ensures the care you need. By prioritizing your comfort and well-being, you support your recovery and enhance your postpartum experience.

Safe Postpartum Exercises for New Moms

Postpartum exercise can be transformative for your recovery and overall well-being. Gentle physical activity offers numerous benefits, including increased energy, improved mood, and accelerated healing. Exercise stimulates the release of endorphins, which help reduce stress and elevate your mood. It also enhances circulation, delivering oxygen and nutrients to tissues for faster recovery. Conversely, prolonged inactivity can slow recovery, increase discomfort, and raise the risk of complications like blood clots. Integrating safe exercises into your daily routine can make a significant difference.

Before starting any exercise routine, wait for medical clearance from your healthcare provider. This is typically around six weeks postpartum but may vary depending on your delivery and recovery. Once cleared, begin with gentle activities like walking and stretching.

Walking is one of the safest and most effective postpartum exercises. It's low-impact and easily adjustable to your fitness level. Start with short, leisurely walks around your home or neighborhood. As you build strength, gradually increase your distance and pace. Walking not only enhances cardiovascular health but also provides a mental break, helping you clear your mind and enjoy fresh air.

Gentle stretching is an excellent way to ease back into physical activity. Simple stretches can help relieve muscle tension, improve flexibility, and promote relaxation. Focus on areas that commonly hold tension, such as the neck, shoulders, and lower back. For instance, a gentle neck stretch involves slowly tilting your head to one side, holding the position for a few seconds, and then repeating on the other side. Gentle yoga can also be highly beneficial. Poses like child's pose and cat-cow stretch are particularly effective for postpartum recovery. Child's pose helps stretch the lower back and hips, while cat-cow stretch promotes spinal flexibility and relieves tension. These exercises can be performed at home with minimal equipment, making them both accessible and convenient.

Pelvic tilts are another simple yet effective exercise for new mothers. This exercise strengthens the abdominal muscles and improves pelvic stability. To perform a pelvic tilt, lie on your back with your knees bent and feet flat on the floor. Tighten your abdominal muscles and press your lower back into the floor, tilting your pelvis upward. Hold the position for a few seconds, then relax and repeat. This exercise can alleviate lower back pain and strengthen your core, which is essential for overall stability and function. Incorporating pelvic tilts into your daily routine can provide significant benefits without requiring much time or effort.

Listening to your body is paramount when it comes to postpartum exercise. Pay close attention to how you feel during and after each activity. Signs of overexertion include pain, excessive fatigue, and increased bleeding. If you experience any of these symptoms, scale back your activity and allow yourself more time to rest. Adjusting your routine is both normal and necessary to ensure a safe recovery. Taking breaks and modifying exercises as needed can help you avoid setbacks and promote a more sustainable approach to physical activity. Remember, it's not about pushing yourself to the limit but rather finding a balance that supports your well-being.

Quick Exercise Routine for New Moms
- **Walking**: Start with a 10-minute walk around your neighborhood, gradually increasing the time and distance as you feel more comfortable.

- **Gentle Yoga**: Practice child's pose and cat-cow stretch for 5-10 minutes to relieve tension and improve flexibility.
- **Pelvic Tilts**: Perform 10-15 repetitions of pelvic tilts, focusing on proper form and breathing.

Incorporating these exercises into your daily routine provides a gentle yet effective way to support postpartum recovery. The key is to start slow, listen to your body, and gradually increase the intensity as you regain strength and confidence. Every small step toward physical activity contributes to your overall health and well-being during this crucial period.

Understanding and Handling Postpartum Bleeding

Postpartum bleeding, also known as lochia, is a normal part of the recovery process after childbirth. This bleeding is your body's way of shedding the extra tissue and blood that supported your pregnancy. It typically lasts several weeks and occurs in three distinct stages.

1. **Lochia Rubra**: During the first few days postpartum, you will experience bright red bleeding that may contain small clots. This stage can be quite heavy, resembling a very heavy menstrual period.
2. **Lochia Serosa**: From about day four to ten, the bleeding will lighten and turn pinkish-brown.
3. **Lochia Alba**: Finally, the discharge becomes yellowish-white and may continue for several weeks.

It's crucial to differentiate between normal and abnormal postpartum bleeding. Normal bleeding should gradually decrease over time. If you find yourself soaking through a maternity pad in less than an hour, this could indicate abnormal bleeding. Other warning signs include passing large clots (bigger than a golf ball), a foul odor from the discharge, or a sudden increase in bleeding after it had started to taper off. Heavy bleeding, known as postpartum hemorrhage, is a medical emergency that requires immediate attention. Symptoms like dizziness, a rapid pulse, or fainting also warrant prompt medical care.

Managing Postpartum Bleeding

Managing postpartum bleeding involves practical strategies to ensure comfort and hygiene:

- **Use Maternity Pads**: These are more absorbent than regular menstrual pads. Change them frequently to prevent infections and maintain hygiene.
- **Avoid Tampons**: Tampons can introduce bacteria and increase the risk of infection.
- **Keep the Perineal Area Clean**: Use a peri bottle filled with warm water to gently cleanse the area after using the bathroom. Pat dry with a clean towel rather than wiping to avoid irritation. Regular showers also help maintain hygiene. Avoid soaking in baths until your healthcare provider gives the go-ahead.
- **Choose Breathable Clothing**: Loose, breathable cotton underwear can help keep the area dry and comfortable.

Knowing When to Seek Medical Attention

It's essential to recognize signs that require medical intervention:

- Heavy bleeding that soaks through a pad in an hour or less.
- A foul odor from the discharge, which could indicate infection.
- Fever, which may signal an infection.

Trust your instincts—if something feels off, consult your healthcare provider immediately.

Many mothers have shared similar experiences, and knowing you're not alone can be reassuring. For instance, Sarah, a first-time mom, was initially worried when she noticed bright red bleeding. However, after discussing it with her doctor and hearing similar stories from other moms, she felt more at ease. Dr. Emily Johnson, an OB-GYN, explains, *"Postpartum bleeding is your body's way of healing and returning to its pre-pregnancy state. It's normal for the bleeding to go through different stages and gradually decrease over time."*

Personal stories and professional reassurance can help normalize the experience and reduce anxiety. Postpartum bleeding is a sign that your body is undergoing the necessary steps for recovery. By managing it effectively and knowing when to seek medical advice, you can focus on your well-being and enjoy precious moments with your new baby.

As you navigate postpartum bleeding, remember that it's a temporary phase. With the right care and attention, your body will heal, and the bleeding will eventually stop. Stay vigilant, practice good hygiene, and don't hesitate to reach out to your healthcare provider if you have any concerns. Your recovery is a journey, and each step brings you closer to feeling like yourself again.

Chapter 3:
Feeding Your Newborn

The first time I held my newborn to breastfeed, I was filled with both excitement and trepidation. Despite reading books and attending classes, when the moment arrived, I felt unprepared. My baby struggled to latch, and I winced in pain. It was then I realized that breastfeeding, while natural, often requires guidance and practice. This chapter aims to demystify the process and provide you with the tools to make feeding your newborn a rewarding experience.

Breastfeeding Basics: Getting the Right Latch
A good latch is the cornerstone of successful breastfeeding. It ensures that your baby receives enough milk and that you remain comfortable. When your baby is properly latched, milk transfer is efficient, keeping your baby satiated and aiding healthy weight gain. Conversely, a poor latch can lead to several issues. One immediate concern is nipple pain and damage, as improper positioning may cause the baby to suck only on the nipple, resulting in soreness or cracks. Over time, a poor latch can also increase the risk of mastitis, a painful infection of the breast tissue. Establishing a good latch from the start can prevent these complications, making breastfeeding more enjoyable for both you and your baby.

Achieving a good latch involves several steps, starting with positioning. Hold your baby tummy-to-tummy with you, ensuring their head is aligned with their body. This alignment helps them open their mouth wide, which is essential for a deep latch. Gently brush your nipple against their upper lip to encourage them to open their mouth. When they do, bring them to your breast, aiming the nipple towards the roof of their mouth. This helps your baby take in a good portion of the areola, not just the nipple. Support your baby's head and shoulders without forcing them, allowing them to latch naturally. The breast should hang naturally, ensuring a deep latch that is comfortable for both of you.

Recognizing a good latch is crucial. When the latch is correct, your baby's mouth will cover most of the areola, not just the nipple. There should be no clicking sounds during feeding, as these can indicate a shallow latch. When your baby releases the nipple, it should appear rounded, not flattened or pinched. Additionally, your baby's lips should flare outward, resembling fish lips, with their chin touching your breast. You may also notice slight movements in their ears as they suck, indicating effective milk transfer.

If breastfeeding is painful or your baby is not gaining weight as expected, it's essential to address these issues. Start by adjusting your baby's position, as even small changes can make a significant difference. Experiment with different breastfeeding holds to find what works best for you both. The cradle hold is a common and comfortable position, where your baby's chest rests against your abdomen, supported by your forearm. The football hold, where you tuck your baby under your arm, can be especially helpful after a C-section or if you have larger breasts. Each position offers unique angles and support, potentially improving the latch.

If adjustments don't resolve the issue, seek help from a lactation consultant. They can observe a feeding session and provide personalized advice. Sometimes, underlying conditions like tongue-tie or lip-tie can affect latching. A professional can diagnose these issues and recommend appropriate interventions. Remember, breastfeeding is a learning process for both you and your baby. With patience, practice, and support, you can overcome challenges and enjoy a successful breastfeeding journey.

Overcoming Common Breastfeeding Challenges
Breastfeeding can be a beautiful experience, but it comes with its share of challenges. One common issue is sore nipples and breast pain. Nipple pain can range from mild discomfort to severe pain that makes breastfeeding unbearable. Applying lanolin cream can soothe and heal cracked nipples. Lanolin is safe for both you and your baby and doesn't need to be wiped off before feeding. Cold compresses are also highly effective, reducing swelling and numbing the area for temporary relief. Use a cold pack or a bag of frozen peas wrapped in a cloth to avoid direct contact with the skin.

Low milk supply is another concern for many new mothers. It's natural to worry about whether your baby is getting enough milk, but several strategies can help boost production. Frequent feeding is one of the most effective methods. Nursing on demand, rather than adhering to a strict schedule, ensures that your baby signals your body to produce more milk. Pumping after feeds can also help stimulate additional milk production. Some foods and supplements, like oatmeal and fenugreek, are believed to increase milk supply, but consult your healthcare provider before starting any new supplement. Engorgement and clogged ducts are other common issues that can cause discomfort. Engorgement occurs when your breasts are overly full, making them hard and painful. Hand-expressing a small amount of milk before feeding can provide relief and make it easier for your baby to latch. Warm compresses before feeding can soften the breast and encourage milk flow, while gentle breast massage, starting from the outer edges and moving toward the nipple, can help clear blockages. If you feel a lump in your breast, it may be a clogged duct. Continue nursing frequently, use warm compresses, and massage the area to alleviate the blockage.

Thrush and mastitis are conditions that can make breastfeeding painful and challenging. Thrush is a yeast infection that can affect both your nipples and your baby's mouth. Symptoms include white patches in your baby's mouth and persistent nipple pain that doesn't improve despite proper latch techniques. Over-the-counter antifungal medications can help, but it's best to consult your healthcare provider for a proper diagnosis and treatment plan. Mastitis, on the other hand, is a bacterial infection that typically results from a clogged duct. Symptoms include fever, chills, and red streaks on the breast. Antibiotics are usually required to treat mastitis, so it's essential to seek medical attention if you suspect you have it.

Recognizing the symptoms of these conditions early is crucial for effective treatment. If you notice white patches in your baby's mouth or ongoing nipple pain, it could be thrush. For mastitis, watch for fever and red, inflamed areas on your breast. Both conditions can make breastfeeding difficult, but with prompt treatment, you can continue nursing your baby and maintaining your milk supply.

Breastfeeding challenges can feel daunting, but you're not alone. Many mothers face these issues, and there are practical solutions to help you overcome them. From applying lanolin cream for sore nipples to using warm compresses for engorgement, these tips can make a significant difference. If you're struggling with low milk supply, frequent feeding and pumping can help boost production. Don't hesitate to seek support from your healthcare provider or a lactation consultant. Breastfeeding is a learning process for both you and your baby, and with time and patience, it can become a rewarding experience for you both.

Bottle-Feeding Tips and Techniques

Bottle-feeding can be a practical and effective way to ensure your baby gets the nutrition they need, whether you are supplementing breastfeeding or using formula. Choosing the right bottle and nipple is the first important step. Bottles come in various shapes and sizes, and nipples have different flow rates. For newborns, a slow-flow nipple is usually best, as it mimics the natural flow of breastfeeding. This can help prevent overfeeding and reduce the risk of choking. As your baby grows and their feeding needs change, you can switch to nipples with faster flow rates. It's also essential to choose bottles that are easy to clean and assemble. Some parents prefer bottles with fewer parts for convenience, while others opt for designs that reduce gas and colic.

Proper sterilization techniques are critical to keeping your baby's bottles free from harmful bacteria. Before the first use, bottles and nipples should be sterilized by boiling them in water for five minutes or using a steam sterilizer. After the initial sterilization, you can wash bottles and nipples in hot, soapy water or in the dishwasher if they are dishwasher-safe. Regular cleaning is essential to keep the feeding equipment hygienic and safe. Be sure to check the nipples for any signs of wear and tear, replacing them as needed.

Introducing the bottle to a breastfed baby can be a smooth transition with the right strategies. Timing is key—it's best to introduce the bottle when your baby is calm and not too

35

hungry. A fussy or overly hungry baby may resist the bottle, making the experience stressful for both of you. Using a slow-flow nipple can help mimic the breastfeeding experience, easing the transition. Start by offering the bottle during a relaxed time, such as after a nap. Allow someone else, like your partner, to give the first bottle, as your baby may associate you with breastfeeding and resist the bottle if you offer it.

Paced bottle-feeding is a method that mimics the natural flow of breastfeeding and helps prevent overfeeding. To practice paced feeding, hold your baby in an upright position. This position allows better control of the flow and reduces the risk of choking. Hold the bottle parallel to the ground and let your baby take a few sucks before gently pulling the bottle back. This pause allows your baby to control the flow and take breaks as needed, similar to breastfeeding. It also helps prevent your baby from swallowing too much air, reducing the chances of gas and discomfort. Be attentive to your baby's cues, such as turning away or slowing down, to know when they've had enough.

Choosing the right bottle-feeding position can make the experience comfortable and promote bonding. The cradle hold is a common position where you hold your baby in your arms, with their head resting in the crook of your elbow. This position allows for eye contact and close physical contact, enhancing bonding. Another effective position is the side-lying position, particularly useful for nighttime feedings or after a C-section. Lie on your side with your baby facing you, supported by your arm. This position can be relaxing and allows you to rest while feeding your baby.

Bottle-feeding offers flexibility and allows other family members to participate in feeding, giving you a much-needed break. It's important to create a calm and relaxed environment during feeding times. This helps your baby feel secure and makes feeding a positive experience. Whether you're exclusively bottle-feeding or combining it with breastfeeding, the key is to find what works best for you and your baby. Every baby is unique, so be patient and open to trying different techniques and positions until you find the perfect fit for both of you.

Estimating Your Baby's Milk Needs

Determining if your baby is getting enough milk can be a common concern for new mothers, whether breastfeeding or bottle-feeding. One reliable indicator is tracking your baby's output. For both breastfed and bottle-fed babies, wet and dirty diapers are clear signs of adequate intake. In the early days, your newborn should produce at least one wet diaper per day of life, increasing to about six to eight wet diapers daily by the end of the first week. Dirty diapers are equally important; expect at least three to four bowel movements each day in the initial weeks. Monitoring these outputs can help reassure you that your baby is getting enough milk.

Tracking your baby's weight gain is another critical method. Regular weight checks, especially in the first few weeks, provide valuable insight into your baby's growth. While most newborns lose some weight initially, they should regain it by about two weeks of age. After this period, a steady weekly weight gain of approximately 5–7 ounces is typical. Regular pediatrician visits for weight monitoring can help confirm that your baby is thriving and receiving adequate nutrition.

Feeding schedules vary depending on your baby's age and developmental stage. During the newborn phase, frequent, smaller feeds are typical, with most newborns feeding every two to three hours—or about eight to twelve times in 24 hours. This frequent feeding ensures they get enough milk and helps stimulate your supply if you're breastfeeding. As your baby grows, feeding intervals may lengthen, particularly at night. Growth spurts—commonly occurring around three weeks, six weeks, and three months—often lead to more frequent feeding. These temporary increases in demand are vital for supporting your baby's rapid development.

Recognizing hunger cues is key to feeding on demand and meeting your baby's needs promptly. Early hunger cues include rooting (turning their head toward your hand or breast) and sucking on their hands or fingers. These subtle signs indicate that your baby is ready to feed. Late hunger cues, such as crying and fussiness, suggest they are already very hungry and may be harder to soothe. Responding to early hunger signals can make feeding smoother and less stressful for both of you.

Adjusting feeding amounts as your baby grows is essential to meet their changing nutritional needs. For bottle-fed babies, start with smaller amounts and gradually increase them as they grow. Watch for signs of fullness or hunger to guide you. A content, relaxed baby who sleeps well and has regular wet and dirty diapers is likely receiving adequate milk. Conversely, signs of dissatisfaction, fussiness, or fewer wet diapers might indicate the need to increase feeding amounts.

During the first few months, your baby's feeding needs will evolve frequently. Being attentive and flexible helps ensure they receive the right amount of milk. Regularly monitor their output, growth, and behavior, and consult your pediatrician for additional guidance and reassurance. Feeding your newborn is a dynamic process, and understanding their cues can help you navigate it confidently.

Pumping and Storing Breast Milk

Pumping breast milk offers numerous benefits and is a valuable practice for many new mothers. A primary reason to pump is to maintain your milk supply. Regular pumping signals your body to continue producing milk, even if you're away from your baby or if they are not nursing as frequently. Pumping also allows others, such as your partner or family members, to feed the baby, giving you much-needed breaks to rest. Additionally, pumping helps you build a milk stash, which can be especially useful when returning to work, ensuring your baby continues to benefit from breast milk even when you're not present.

Choosing the right breast pump is crucial for effective and comfortable pumping. Pumps come in different types, each with unique features. Manual pumps are hand-operated, more affordable, and portable, making them ideal for occasional use. Electric pumps, however, are more efficient and save time, especially for regular pumping. Within the electric category, single pumps extract milk from one breast at a time, while double pumps allow simultaneous pumping from both breasts, significantly reducing pumping time. When selecting a pump, consider your pumping frequency, budget, and personal preferences.

Effective pumping involves more than just having the right equipment. Creating a comfortable environment is essential. Find a quiet, relaxing space where you can sit comfortably without distractions. Stimulate letdown by applying warm compresses to your breasts or gently massaging them before pumping to encourage milk flow. When you're ready, attach the pump and adjust the suction and speed settings. Start with a lower suction setting and gradually increase it to a comfortable level. Pumping should not be painful—if you experience discomfort, reduce the suction or adjust the flange positioning.

Storing Breast Milk Properly

Proper storage of breast milk ensures it remains safe and nutritious for your baby. Use containers specifically designed for breast milk, such as storage bags or bottles. Label each container with the date and time of expression to track its freshness. Freshly pumped milk can be stored in the refrigerator for up to four days. For longer storage, freezing is a reliable option. Breast milk can be stored in a freezer for up to six months or in a deep freezer for up to twelve months. When freezing, leave some space at the top of the container to allow for expansion.

Thawing and warming breast milk require care to preserve its nutrients. To thaw frozen milk, place the container in the refrigerator overnight or run it under warm water. Avoid using a microwave, as it can create hot spots and destroy some of the milk's beneficial properties. Once thawed, warm the milk by placing the container in a bowl of warm water. Swirl the milk gently to mix any separated fat. Test the temperature before feeding your baby by placing a few drops on your wrist; it should feel lukewarm, not hot.

Pumping and storing breast milk can be a rewarding process that offers flexibility and support for both you and your baby. By understanding the benefits of pumping, choosing the right equipment, and following proper techniques, you can make the experience more efficient and comfortable. Proper storage ensures your baby continues to receive the nutritional benefits of breast milk, even when you're not present. This practice not only supports your milk supply but also allows others to help with feeding, giving you opportunities to rest and recharge.

Transitioning Between Breast and Bottle
Transitioning between breast and bottle is a decision many mothers face for various reasons. A common reason is returning to work. Balancing a career and breastfeeding can be challenging, and introducing a bottle allows you to maintain your milk supply while being away from your baby. It also enables your partner to participate in feeding, fostering a deeper bond with the baby. Sharing this responsibility can relieve some of the pressure on you and provide much-needed breaks. Another reason for transitioning is managing milk supply issues; supplementing with a bottle can help ensure your baby continues to receive adequate nutrition.

Making the transition from breast to bottle requires a gradual approach to ease the change for both you and your baby. Start by introducing the bottle slowly. Choose a time when your baby is calm and content, rather than very hungry or fussy. Initially, use breast milk in the bottle to make the experience more familiar. This can help your baby accept the bottle without resistance. Offering the bottle at different times of the day can also help your baby adjust. For instance, start with one bottle feeding per day and gradually increase as your baby becomes more comfortable.

Challenges may arise during this transition, but they can be managed with patience and persistence. Nipple confusion is a common issue where the baby struggles to switch between breast and bottle. To minimize this, offer the bottle at specific times, such as when you are not present. This helps your baby learn to accept both feeding methods. Resistance to the bottle is another potential challenge. Experimenting with different bottle types and nipple shapes can help find one your baby prefers. Babies often have unique preferences, so some trial and error may be needed.

Flexibility and patience are essential for a smooth transition. Every baby is different, and what works for one may not work for another. Be patient and give your baby time to adjust. If they initially refuse the bottle, avoid forcing it. Instead, try again later or the next day. Observe your baby's preferences and adapt your approach as needed. Some babies may take longer to get used to the bottle, while others adjust quickly. Your patience and flexibility will make the process smoother for both of you.

In summary, transitioning between breast and bottle is a common need for many mothers due to factors such as returning to work, involving a partner in feeding, and managing milk supply. Gradual introduction, using breast milk initially, and offering the bottle at specific times can ease the process. Challenges like nipple confusion and resistance can be addressed with patience and by trying different bottles. By remaining flexible and understanding, you can make this transition a positive experience for both you and your baby.

Chapter 4:
Establishing Sleep Routines

When my youngest daughter was born, I vividly remember how elusive sleep became. Nights blurred into days, and the fatigue was overwhelming. It wasn't until I realized the importance of creating an optimal sleep environment that we all began to get the rest we needed. The right setting can make a significant difference in promoting better sleep for both your baby and yourself.

Creating a Sleep-Friendly Environment
A conducive sleep environment is fundamental for helping your baby sleep well. The surroundings can influence the quality of sleep and the ease with which your baby falls asleep. One of the most effective ways to create a sleep-friendly environment is by ensuring the room is dark and quiet. Babies are often sensitive to light and noise, which can disturb their sleep. Blackout curtains are an excellent investment for this purpose. They block out external light, creating a dark and soothing environment that mimics nighttime, even during the day. According to **Sleepout Curtains**, blackout curtains also offer additional benefits like noise reduction and energy efficiency, making them a multifunctional addition to your nursery.

Choosing a comfortable crib or bassinet that adheres to safe sleep guidelines is another critical step. The crib should have a firm mattress and a fitted sheet, with no loose bedding, pillows, or stuffed toys, as these items can pose a risk of suffocation. The **American Academy of Pediatrics** recommends placing your baby on their back to sleep, as this position reduces the risk of sudden infant death syndrome (SIDS). A safe sleep space can give you peace of mind and help your baby sleep more soundly.

Temperature regulation is another essential factor in creating a sleep-friendly environment. The ideal room temperature for a baby is between 68°F and 72°F (20°C to 22°C), according to **Healthline**. Maintaining this temperature range helps prevent overheating, which has been linked to SIDS. Using a fan can help circulate air and keep the room cool, while a heater can be useful during colder months. Always ensure that fans and heaters are placed safely out of reach and are not blowing directly on your baby. An indoor thermometer can help you monitor the room temperature and make adjustments as needed.

White noise can be a game-changer for soothing and settling your baby. It mimics the sounds your baby heard in the womb, providing a calming effect that can help them fall asleep and stay asleep. White noise machines offer various sound options, including white, pink, and brown noise, each providing different levels of noise masking. The **LectroFan EVO** is a highly recommended option that offers 22 different sounds and is compact and travel-friendly. If you prefer not to use a machine, alternatives like white noise apps or household items such as fans or humidifiers can also be effective.

Minimizing distractions in the sleep environment is equally important. Remove stimulating toys and decorations from the crib, as these can be visually distracting and keep your baby awake. Limit light exposure by using dim nightlights, which provide just enough illumination for you to check on your baby without disturbing their sleep. A calm and uncluttered environment helps signal to your baby that it's time to sleep.

Sleep Environment Checklist
- **Dark, quiet room**: Use blackout curtains to block out light and reduce noise.
- **Comfortable crib or bassinet**: Ensure it meets safe sleep guidelines with a firm mattress and no loose bedding.
- **Temperature regulation**: Maintain a room temperature of 68°F to 72°F using fans or heaters as needed.
- **White noise**: Consider a white noise machine or alternative options to soothe your baby.
- **Minimize distractions**: Remove stimulating toys and use dim nightlights.

Creating a sleep-friendly environment takes some effort, but the rewards are well worth it. By addressing factors such as light, noise, temperature, and distractions, you can help your baby establish healthy sleep patterns. This not only benefits your baby but also contributes to a more restful and manageable routine for you.

Sample Sleep Schedules for Newborns
Establishing a sleep schedule for your baby can feel like a daunting task, but it's incredibly helpful for both you and your little one. Newborns, those precious bundles aged 0–3 months, typically need frequent naps throughout the day. Their sleep cycles are short, and they often wake every two to three hours, whether it's day or night. A typical schedule for a newborn might involve waking up around 7 a.m., followed by a feed and some brief awake time. This pattern of sleep, feeding, and wakefulness continues throughout the day, with naps lasting anywhere from 30 minutes to two hours. During the night, aim for longer stretches of sleep, but expect to wake up for

feedings every few hours.

As your baby grows and enters the 3–6 month stage, their sleep patterns start to shift. Infants this age usually take fewer naps during the day, but these naps tend to be longer. You might find that your baby settles into a more predictable routine with three to four naps, each lasting about one to two hours. During the night, many infants begin to sleep for longer stretches, perhaps waking only once or twice for feedings. A typical day might start around 7 a.m. with a wake-up and feed, followed by a morning nap around 9 a.m. Another nap might occur in the early afternoon, with a shorter nap in the late afternoon. Bedtime often falls between 7 and 8 p.m., allowing for a longer nighttime sleep.

The concept of wake windows is crucial in establishing a successful sleep schedule. Wake windows refer to the amount of time your baby can comfortably stay awake between naps. For newborns, these windows are quite short, often just 45 minutes to an hour. As your baby grows, the wake windows gradually lengthen. By the time your baby is 3–6 months old, they might be able to stay awake for 1.5 to 2 hours between naps. Keeping an eye on these wake windows helps prevent overtiredness, which can make it harder for your baby to fall asleep and stay asleep. Signs of overstimulation include fussiness, difficulty settling, and rubbing their eyes. Recognizing these cues can help you adjust the schedule to better meet your baby's needs.

Adapting sleep schedules as your baby grows involves gradual changes. Start by extending wake windows by 10–15 minutes every few days, observing how your baby responds. If they handle the longer awake time well, continue to slowly lengthen it. Always monitor your baby's cues to ensure they are not becoming overtired. Adjusting nap lengths and times as needed can help fine-tune the schedule. For example, if your baby consistently wakes up early from an afternoon nap, consider moving it slightly later or earlier to see if it helps.

Consistency is the cornerstone of establishing a successful sleep routine. Maintaining regular bedtime rituals helps signal to your baby that it's time to wind down and get ready for sleep. A calming routine might include a warm bath, a soothing story, and some gentle lullabies. These activities can create a sense of security and help your baby transition from wakefulness to sleep. Daily routines are equally important. Consistent feeding times and playtimes help regulate your baby's internal clock, making it easier for them to predict what comes next. Over time, this consistency helps establish a rhythm that supports healthy sleep habits.

Creating a solid sleep schedule involves understanding your baby's developmental stage and adjusting as they grow. For newborns, frequent naps and short wake windows are the norm, while infants begin to consolidate sleep with fewer, longer naps. Paying attention to wake windows and signs of overstimulation can help you fine-tune the schedule. Gradual adjustments and consistent routines are key to helping your baby develop healthy sleep habits.

Sleep Training Techniques
Introducing sleep training can feel overwhelming, but understanding different methods can help you find the best approach for your family. The Ferber method, developed by Dr. Richard Ferber, involves progressive waiting. This technique aims to teach babies to self-soothe by allowing them to cry for predetermined intervals before offering comfort. On the first night, you might start with three-minute intervals,

gradually increasing to five and then ten minutes. Each subsequent night, the intervals lengthen, helping your baby learn to fall asleep independently. This method is often effective, yielding faster results, but it does involve periods of crying, which can be challenging for some parents to endure.

The Chair method, also known as gradual withdrawal, takes a more step-by-step approach. You start by placing a chair next to your baby's crib, offering comfort and reassurance without picking them up. Each night, you move the chair further away until you're eventually outside the room. This method requires patience and consistency but can be less distressing for both you and your baby compared to more abrupt methods. While it might take longer to see results, the gradual nature of this approach can make the transition smoother.

For those who prefer a gentler approach, the No Tears method offers a gradual and comforting way to help your baby sleep. This method involves soothing techniques such as patting, shushing, and gentle rocking, gradually decreasing your presence and assistance over time. You might start by rocking your baby until they are almost asleep, then transitioning to patting and shushing in the crib. Over time, you reduce the amount of intervention needed, allowing your baby to learn to fall asleep on their own. The No Tears method minimizes crying, making it more manageable for parents who find it difficult to let their baby cry. However, it often takes longer to achieve consistent sleep patterns.

Each method has its pros and cons. The Ferber method can yield quicker results, but the crying involved can be hard for both parents and baby. The Chair method offers a middle ground with a gradual approach, but it requires a significant time investment and consistency. The No Tears method is the gentlest, reducing stress and crying, but it demands a lot of patience as progress can be slow. Understanding these nuances can help you choose the method that aligns best with your parenting style and your baby's temperament.

Implementing these techniques requires a detailed plan. For the Ferber method, start by establishing a bedtime routine that includes calming activities like a bath and story-time. Place your baby in the crib drowsy but awake, then leave the room. If your baby cries, wait for the predetermined interval before briefly returning to soothe without picking them up. Gradually increase the intervals over several nights. The Chair method involves a similar bedtime routine, but you stay in the room, sitting in a chair by the crib. Each night, move the chair further away until you're out of the room. With the No Tears method, continue your bedtime routine but focus on reducing your intervention gradually. Start with rocking until drowsy, then transition to patting and shushing in the crib, slowly decreasing your presence over time.

Consistency and patience are paramount in sleep training. Setting realistic expectations helps you stay committed. Understand that sleep training is a process and that setbacks may occur. Keeping a sleep diary can be immensely helpful. Track your baby's sleep patterns, noting what works and what doesn't. This record can provide valuable insights and help you adjust your approach as needed. Remember, every baby is different, and what works for one might not work for another. Patience is essential. There will be nights when progress seems slow or nonexistent. Trust in the process and stay consistent. Your dedication will pay off, leading to better sleep for both your baby and yourself.

Understanding Sleep Regressions

Sleep regressions are phenomena that can leave you feeling puzzled and exhausted. They typically occur at certain stages in your baby's development, often around 4 months, 8-10 months, and 18 months. These periods can last anywhere from two to six weeks, during which your baby's previously established sleep patterns may suddenly change. You might find that your baby, who was sleeping through the night, now wakes up multiple times or has difficulty settling down. Understanding what triggers these regressions can help you navigate them more effectively.

The causes of sleep regressions are usually tied to significant developmental milestones. For instance, around the 4-month mark, your baby undergoes a cognitive leap that increases their awareness of the world around them. This newfound awareness can make it harder for them to settle down to sleep as their brain processes all these exciting new stimuli. Similarly, physical milestones like crawling and walking, which often occur around 8-10 months and 18 months, can disrupt sleep. Your baby might wake up to practice their new skills or because their body is adjusting to these changes. Recognizing that these disruptions are a normal part of development can provide some comfort during these challenging times.

Managing sleep regressions requires a blend of consistency and flexibility. Maintaining your baby's regular sleep routines is crucial. Consistency helps signal to your baby that it's time to sleep, even if their sleep patterns are currently erratic. Stick to your bedtime rituals, whether it's a warm bath, a soothing story, or quiet time in a dimly lit room. These routines provide a sense of security and can help your baby settle down. However, you might need to offer additional comfort during these periods. Extra soothing, whether through gentle rocking, patting, or simply being present, can help reassure your baby.

It's okay to provide more comfort than usual, knowing that this phase is temporary.

Reassuring yourself that sleep regressions are normal and will pass is just as important as soothing your baby. Many parents experience this, and sharing stories can be incredibly comforting. For instance, one mother, Emily, shared how her 4-month-old suddenly started waking every two hours. She was at her wit's end until she spoke with her pediatrician and learned about sleep regressions. Knowing it was a temporary phase helped her cope better. Pediatricians often reassure parents that these regressions, though challenging, are a sign that their baby is developing as expected. Dr. Sarah Mitchell, a pediatric sleep consultant, often tells parents, "These regressions are your baby's way of telling you they're growing and changing. It's a frustrating but positive sign of development."

Recognizing that these phases are temporary can help you maintain your sanity. Sleep regressions usually last between two and six weeks. While this might feel like an eternity when you're in the thick of it, knowing there's an end in sight can be a huge relief. It's also helpful to remember that these phases are a sign of your baby's growth and development. They are learning, adapting, and becoming more aware of their surroundings. This perspective can make the sleepless nights a bit more bearable.

During these periods, it's important to take care of yourself as well. Try to rest when your baby sleeps, and don't hesitate to ask for help from your partner, family, or friends. Sharing the load can make a significant difference in how you cope with sleep regressions. Taking care of your well-being allows you to be more patient and effective in comforting your baby.

In conclusion, sleep regressions are a normal part of your baby's development. They often occur around 4 months, 8-10 months, and 18 months and can last for a few weeks. These regressions are triggered by cognitive and physical milestones, making it harder for your baby to settle down. Managing these periods involves maintaining consistent sleep routines and offering extra comfort. Remember, these phases are temporary and a sign of healthy development. Seek support from other parents and professionals to navigate this challenging but normal part of parenthood.

Co-Sleeping: Pros and Cons

Co-sleeping is a topic that brings out strong opinions. On one hand, it offers several benefits that can make those early months a bit easier. One of the most significant advantages is the convenience it provides for nighttime feedings. If you're breastfeeding, having your baby close by means you don't have to get up and walk to another room multiple times a night. This setup can make the process smoother and less disruptive for both you and your baby. You can feed your baby and then settle them back to sleep with minimal effort, allowing everyone to get back to sleep more quickly.

Increased bonding is another compelling reason many parents choose to co-sleep. The physical closeness can enhance the emotional bond between you and your baby. Babies often find comfort in the presence of their parents, which can help them feel more secure and settle down more easily. The skin-to-skin contact during co-sleeping can also be soothing, helping to regulate your baby's body temperature and heart rate. This closeness can make nighttime wakings feel less like a chore and more like an opportunity for cuddles and connection.

However, co-sleeping comes with its own set of risks and safety concerns. One of the primary concerns is the increased risk of sudden infant death syndrome (SIDS). The American Academy of Pediatrics advises against bed-sharing due to potential hazards like suffocation, entrapment, and overheating. It's crucial to follow safety guidelines if you choose to co-sleep. Ensure that the mattress is firm and free of loose bedding, pillows, or soft toys that could pose a risk. Never co-sleep on a couch or armchair, as these surfaces are particularly dangerous. Instead, consider room-sharing, where your baby sleeps in a separate crib or bassinet in your room. This arrangement allows you to keep your baby close while adhering to safer sleep practices.

For parents who want the benefits of closeness without the risks associated with bed-sharing, bedside sleepers can be an excellent alternative. These are specially designed cribs that attach securely to your bed, allowing your baby to sleep in their own safe space while still being within arm's reach. Bedside sleepers can make nighttime feedings more convenient and provide the comfort of closeness without the dangers of bed-sharing. Room-sharing is another viable option. Setting up a crib or bassinet in your room offers the benefits of co-sleeping while ensuring a safer sleep environment. This setup allows you to respond quickly to your baby's needs and provides peace of mind knowing they are close by.

Transitioning your baby out of co-sleeping and into their own sleep space can be a gradual process. Start by introducing naps in the new sleep space to help your baby get used to it. Gradually increase the amount of time they spend sleeping there. Creating a comfortable and familiar sleep environment can ease this transition. Use items your baby associates with sleep, such as a favorite blanket or a familiar bedtime toy.

Consistent routines, like a calming bedtime ritual, can also help your baby adjust to the new sleep space. This gradual approach can make the transition smoother for both you and your baby, reducing stress and promoting better sleep.

Co-sleeping offers various benefits, such as easier night feedings and increased bonding, but it also comes with risks that need to be carefully managed. Alternatives like bedside sleepers and room-sharing provide safer options while maintaining the closeness that many parents and babies find comforting. Transitioning out of co-sleeping requires patience and a gradual approach, but with consistent routines and familiar items, you can help your baby adjust to their own sleep space effectively.

Dealing with Night Wakings

Night wakings are a common and often frustrating aspect of parenting. Understanding the reasons behind your baby's nocturnal awakenings can help you address them more effectively. One of the most frequent causes of night waking is hunger, especially during growth spurts. Babies grow rapidly, and their nutritional needs can spike suddenly, leaving them hungry more often than usual. During these periods, your baby might wake up more frequently for feedings, which is entirely normal. Another reason for night wakings is discomfort. Teething can cause sore gums, making it hard for your baby to sleep soundly. Similarly, illnesses like colds or ear infections can disrupt sleep. Watch for signs of discomfort, such as fussiness, tugging at the ears, or drooling more than usual.

Developmental milestones are another factor that can cause night wakings. As your baby learns new skills like rolling over, sitting up, or crawling, their sleep might be disrupted. These milestones are exciting but can be overwhelming for a baby's developing brain, leading to increased wakefulness at night. It's important to remember that these phases are temporary and often accompanied by periods of significant growth and learning.

When your baby wakes up at night, soothing and settling them can help everyone get back to sleep more quickly. Gentle rocking in a rocking chair can be incredibly calming. The rhythmic motion mimics the movements your baby felt in the womb, providing a sense of security. Sometimes, a quick feed is all that's needed to settle your baby back to sleep. Decide when to offer a night feed based on your baby's hunger cues and age. For younger infants, frequent night feedings are normal, whereas older babies might not need to feed as often. If a diaper change is necessary, keep it quick and quiet. Use dim lighting and avoid stimulating interactions to help your baby transition back to sleep smoothly.

Encouraging your baby to self-soothe is an important skill that can help reduce night wakings over time. Gradual reduction of assistance, also known as fading techniques, can be effective. Start by providing plenty of comfort and slowly reduce your involvement over time. For example, if you usually rock your baby to sleep, try reducing the time you spend rocking each night. Introduce a comfort object, such as a small blanket or a soft toy, to provide additional reassurance. Ensure the object is safe and suitable for your baby's age. A lovey can become a source of comfort and help your baby learn to fall back asleep independently.

Managing your own sleep is equally important. Napping when your baby naps can help you catch up on rest. It might feel like there's always something else you could be doing, but prioritizing sleep will make you more effective in all your tasks.

Sharing night duties with your partner can also make a big difference. Alternating who gets up with the baby allows both parents to get more uninterrupted sleep. Communication is key to making this arrangement work smoothly. Discuss your schedules and preferences to find a system that works for both of you.

Dealing with night wakings requires understanding the root causes and employing strategies to soothe and settle your baby. Hunger, discomfort, and developmental milestones are common reasons for night wakings. Gentle rocking, quick feeds, and diaper changes can help settle your baby. Encouraging self-soothing through gradual reduction of assistance and introducing a comfort object can promote independent sleep. Remember to take care of your own sleep needs by napping when your baby naps and sharing night duties with your partner. These strategies can help make night wakings more manageable and lead to better sleep for everyone.

Navigating the world of baby sleep can feel overwhelming, but understanding the underlying reasons and employing effective strategies can make a significant difference. As you continue to support your baby's sleep, remember that each phase brings new challenges and milestones. In the next chapter, we'll explore the essentials of newborn care, offering practical tips and insights to help you feel more confident in your parenting journey.

Chapter 5:
Newborn Care Essentials

When I first held my son and looked into his eyes, I was struck by the overwhelming responsibility of caring for this tiny human. Every cry and every movement seemed like a mystery waiting to be solved. Understanding what your baby needs can feel like deciphering a secret code, but learning to interpret their cues is a skill that grows with time and practice. These little signals are your baby's way of communicating with you, and recognizing them is crucial for building trust and ensuring their well-being.

Interpreting Baby Cues
Baby cues are essential for establishing trust and security between you and your newborn. When you respond promptly to your baby's needs, you reinforce their sense of safety and comfort. This responsiveness helps your baby learn that they can rely on you, fostering a secure attachment vital for their emotional development. Recognizing and responding to these cues also ensures that your baby's needs are met promptly, whether they are hungry, tired, or uncomfortable.

Babies use a variety of cues to communicate their needs. Hunger cues are among the most common and easily recognizable. When your baby is hungry, they may root—turning their head towards your breast or hand—or suck on their hands. These early signs indicate that it's time for a feeding. If you wait until they start crying, it might be harder to calm them, so catching these cues early can make feeding times smoother. Sleep cues are another set of signals to watch for. Your baby might rub their eyes, yawn, or become fussier than usual. These signs suggest that they are ready for a nap. Discomfort cues, such as arching their back, crying, or squirming, indicate that something is bothering them. This could be a dirty diaper, gas, or simply a need for a change in position.

Responding to these cues appropriately can make a world of difference. When you notice hunger cues, offer a feeding. Whether you are breastfeeding or bottle-feeding, responding quickly ensures your baby gets the nourishment they need without becoming overly distressed. For sleep cues, try swaddling your baby to provide a sense of security or gently rocking them to help them settle down. If your baby shows signs of discomfort, check their diaper, burp them, or adjust their position to see if that provides relief. Sometimes, just holding and comforting your baby can make them feel better. Understanding and accurately interpreting baby cues can lead to a more content and healthy baby. When you respond to their needs promptly, you reduce the likelihood of prolonged crying and fussiness, which can be stressful for both you and your baby. This responsiveness also enhances the bond between you and your baby, as they learn to trust that you will care for them. This secure attachment lays the foundation for their emotional and social development, helping them grow into confident and well-adjusted individuals.

Learning your baby's cues is an ongoing process. Each baby is unique, and their signals may vary. Over time, you will become more attuned to their specific ways of communicating. The more you practice, the more confident you will become in understanding and responding to their needs. This confidence will not only make you feel more competent as a parent but also contribute to your baby's overall well-being.

Bath Time Basics

Bath time isn't just about keeping your baby clean; it's also a wonderful opportunity for bonding. Regular baths help maintain your newborn's hygiene, keeping their skin healthy and free from irritants. But beyond cleanliness, bath time can be a calming and enjoyable experience for both you and your baby. The warm water and gentle touch create a soothing environment, allowing you to connect and engage with your baby in a unique way. It's a time when you can focus solely on them, away from the distractions of daily life, fostering a sense of security and closeness.

Before you begin, it's important to gather all the necessary supplies. You'll need a baby bathtub or a basin, mild baby soap, a soft washcloth, a cup for rinsing, and a towel. Fill the baby bathtub with just a few inches of warm water, making sure the temperature is between 98°F and 100°F. You can test it using your wrist or elbow; it should feel warm but not hot. Once everything is ready, undress your baby and wrap them in a towel to keep them warm.

Supporting your baby's head and neck is crucial during the bath. Gently lower them into the water, keeping one hand under their head for support. Use your other hand to wash them, starting from the top and working your way down. Begin by using a damp washcloth to clean their face, being careful around the eyes and ears. Next, wash their body with mild baby soap, paying attention to the folds of their skin where dirt and milk can accumulate. Use the cup to gently pour water over their body for rinsing, ensuring the soap is completely washed off. Finally, wash their hair with a small amount of baby shampoo, rinsing carefully to avoid getting water in their eyes. Safety is paramount during bath time. Never leave your baby unattended, even for a moment. If you need to step away, wrap them in a towel and take them with you. To prevent slipping, use a non-slip mat in the baby bathtub or basin. Always test the water temperature before placing your baby in the tub to ensure it's safe. These precautions help ensure that bath time remains a safe and enjoyable experience for both you and your baby.

To make bath time more enjoyable, consider incorporating some fun elements. Soft, waterproof toys like rubber ducks or bath books can keep your baby entertained and make the experience more interactive. Singing or talking to your baby during the bath can also create a soothing atmosphere. Babies love the sound of your voice, and it can help keep them calm and engaged. Make sure to smile and maintain eye contact, reinforcing the bond between you.

Bath time is also an excellent opportunity to establish a bedtime routine. The warm water can help relax your baby, making it easier for them to settle down for the night. After the bath, gently dry your baby with a soft towel, paying close attention to the folds of their skin. Applying a gentle moisturizer can keep their skin soft and hydrated. Dress them in comfortable pajamas, and consider incorporating a soothing activity, such as reading a short story or singing a lullaby.

Creating a positive bath time experience can lay the foundation for a lifetime of healthy hygiene habits and strengthen the bond between you and your baby. Each bath is an opportunity to connect, engage, and create lasting memories. Whether it's the joy of splashing in the water or the comfort of your gentle touch, bath time can become one of the most cherished parts of your day with your newborn.

Diapering 101: Cloth vs. Disposable

Choosing between cloth and disposable diapers can feel like a significant decision, but understanding the pros and cons of each can help you make an informed choice.

Cloth diapers are often praised for their cost-effectiveness and environmental benefits. While the initial investment in cloth diapers is higher, they are generally more economical in the long run. Because they are reusable, they contribute less waste to landfills, making them a more environmentally friendly option. Many parents also find that cloth diapers are gentler on their baby's skin, reducing the likelihood of diaper rash. However, they do require more frequent changes due to lower absorbency and can result in increased laundry, leading to higher water and electricity usage. Cleaning and managing cloth diapers can also be labor-intensive, which may not suit every family's lifestyle.

Disposable diapers, on the other hand, offer unmatched convenience. They feature attached fastening strips, making them easy to use, especially when you're on the go. Their high absorbency means fewer daily diaper changes, which can be a lifesaver during busy days. Additionally, disposable diapers are available in various sizes and designs to suit different needs. However, they can be more expensive over time, and some babies may develop skin irritations from the materials used. Moreover, disposable diapers contribute significantly to landfill waste, raising environmental concerns.

When it comes to the actual process of diapering, each type has specific techniques:

- **Cloth diapers**: Lay the diaper flat and fold it according to the type you're using (e.g., prefolded or all-in-one). Place the diaper under your baby, ensuring the back part reaches their waist. Fold the front part up and secure it with fasteners, ensuring a snug but not tight fit. Check around the legs and waistband to prevent leaks.

- **Disposable diapers**: Open the diaper and place it under your baby, ensuring the back part with the adhesive strips is at waist level. Bring the front part up between their legs and secure the adhesive tabs at the front, checking for gaps around the legs and waistband.

Preventing and treating diaper rash is a common concern. Frequent diaper changes are key to keeping your baby's skin dry and healthy. Aim to change the diaper as soon as it becomes wet or soiled. Applying a thin layer of diaper rash cream during each change can create a protective barrier on the skin. Allowing your baby's bottom to air out occasionally is also beneficial. Letting them go diaper-free for short periods helps keep the area dry and reduces the risk of rash.

Choosing the right diaper size is essential for your baby's comfort and to prevent leaks. Diapers that are too tight can cause discomfort and leave marks on their skin, while loose diapers can lead to leaks. Check the fit around the legs and waistband to ensure there are no gaps. As your baby grows, adjust the size as needed. Most diaper brands provide weight guidelines on their packaging to help you choose the right size. Handling diapering with confidence comes with practice and understanding your baby's needs. Whether you choose cloth or disposable diapers, the key is to stay attentive to your baby's comfort and hygiene. Frequent changes, proper fit, and preventive measures can make diapering smoother and more manageable. Each diaper change is also an opportunity to check in with your baby and ensure they are comfortable and content.

Handling Common Baby Ailments

Newborns, delicate and new to the world, often experience a range of common ailments that can be distressing for both the baby and the parents.

One of the most challenging issues is **colic**, characterized by excessive crying and fussiness. Colic typically peaks around six weeks of age and can last until the baby is about three to four months old. While the exact cause of colic isn't known, it's often attributed to digestive discomfort or an immature nervous system.

To soothe a colicky baby:
- Try using a **colic hold**, where you hold the baby face down along your forearm, supporting their chin in your hand.
- Gentle rocking or swaying can help calm them.
- Some parents find that white noise or a warm bath provides relief.

It's important to remain calm and patient, as your baby can sense your stress.

Jaundice is a common condition in newborns, characterized by a yellowing of the skin and eyes due to high levels of bilirubin in the blood. It is more prevalent in preterm babies and typically appears within the first few days after birth. Ensuring adequate feeding is crucial, as frequent feedings help flush out bilirubin through the baby's stools. Mild jaundice often resolves on its own, but exposing your baby to natural sunlight for short periods can aid in reducing bilirubin levels. Place your baby near a sunny window for about 10 to 15 minutes several times a day, but always supervise closely to avoid overheating. If jaundice persists or worsens, consult your pediatrician for further evaluation and possible treatment, such as phototherapy.

Thrush, another common ailment in newborns, appears as white patches in the mouth and on the tongue. It is caused by a yeast infection from the Candida fungus and can make feeding uncomfortable for your baby. To manage thrush, gently clean your baby's mouth with a damp cloth after feedings. Regularly sterilize bottles and pacifiers to prevent the spread of infection. Consult your doctor for antifungal medication, which may be prescribed for both you and your baby if you are breastfeeding, as the infection can be passed back and forth.

Knowing when to seek medical care is vital for your baby's health. Persistent high fever, difficulty breathing, and severe rashes or skin changes are all signs that require immediate evaluation. A fever higher than 100.4°F (38°C) in a baby younger than three months is considered a medical emergency. If your baby is struggling to breathe or shows signs of respiratory distress, such as rapid breathing or grunting, seek help immediately. Severe rashes, especially those that blister or cause significant discomfort, also warrant prompt medical attention.

Regular pediatric check-ups are essential to monitor your baby's growth and development and to stay up-to-date with vaccinations. Following the recommended immunization schedule protects your baby from serious illnesses. Practicing good hygiene, such as washing your hands before handling your baby and keeping their environment clean, can help prevent infections. Ensuring your baby gets enough rest, proper nutrition, and a safe, clean environment lays the foundation for their well-being.

While common baby ailments can be stressful, having the right knowledge and taking proactive steps can make a significant difference. Understanding conditions like colic, jaundice, and thrush equips you to respond promptly and provide the care your baby needs. Practical solutions—such as using a colic hold for excessive crying, frequent feedings and sunlight exposure for jaundice, and cleaning your baby's mouth for thrush—help address these issues effectively. Recognizing when to seek medical care and prioritizing routine check-ups and immunizations further ensures your baby's health. With attentive care and informed responses, you can navigate these challenges confidently, providing comfort and support to your baby.

Safe Babywearing Techniques
Babywearing is a wonderful practice that offers numerous benefits for both you and your baby. Carrying your baby close allows them to hear your heartbeat, feel your warmth, and smell your scent, fostering a sense of security and trust. This physical closeness strengthens your bond while also being highly convenient. Babywearing keeps your hands free, making it easier to manage daily tasks while caring for your newborn.
Selecting the right baby carrier is essential for both safety and comfort. Options include wraps, slings, and structured carriers. Wraps are versatile pieces of fabric that can be tied in various ways to create a snug fit. Slings, which consist of a loop of fabric worn over one shoulder, are easy to use for quick trips. Structured carriers feature padded straps and buckles, offering more support and ease of use. Look for carriers with safety features such as head and neck support, adjustable straps, and soft, breathable materials.

Proper positioning is critical while babywearing. Your baby's head and neck should always be supported, with their chin off their chest to ensure clear airways. A simple guideline is the "close enough to kiss" rule—your baby's head should be close enough to your mouth for you to kiss the top of their head. Check regularly to ensure their back is straight and their hips are in an "M" position, with knees higher than their bottom. This position supports healthy hip development and ensures comfort.

Choose carrying positions based on your baby's age and your preference. For newborns, the front carry is ideal, with your baby facing inward close to your chest. As your baby gains better head control, the hip carry allows them to observe their surroundings while staying close to you. For older infants who can sit unassisted, the back carry distributes their weight evenly across your shoulders and back, making it more comfortable for longer periods.

Babywearing is not only practical but also enhances the emotional connection between you and your baby. The constant physical contact helps soothe and calm your baby, reducing crying and promoting a sense of well-being. It also allows you to be more attuned to your baby's needs, enabling you to quickly respond to their cues and provide comfort. Whether you use a wrap, sling, or structured carrier, the key is finding what works best for you and your baby. With the right carrier and proper techniques, babywearing can be a rewarding and enjoyable experience for both of you.

Tummy Time: Importance and Tips

Tummy time is a small but crucial part of your baby's daily routine that can significantly impact their development. By placing your baby on their stomach while they are awake, you help them strengthen their neck and shoulder muscles. This is vital as it lays the foundation for future milestones like rolling over, sitting up, and crawling. When your baby pushes up on their arms, they develop the strength and coordination needed for these physical activities. Additionally, tummy time helps prevent flat head syndrome, a condition where the back of a baby's head becomes flattened due to prolonged time spent lying on their back. By incorporating tummy time, you promote a more natural and healthy shape for their developing skull.

Starting tummy time early is key to making it a regular part of your baby's routine. You can begin tummy time from birth, even if it's just for a few minutes each day. Place your baby on a soft, flat surface, like a play mat or a blanket on the floor. Always supervise your baby during tummy time to ensure their safety. Initially, short sessions of about one to two minutes are sufficient. As your baby grows stronger and more comfortable, gradually extend these sessions to 10–15 minutes, several times a day. Over time, your baby will build the strength and endurance needed for longer periods of tummy time.

Making tummy time enjoyable can help your baby look forward to these sessions. Use colorful toys and interesting objects to capture their attention and encourage them to lift their head and reach out. Placing a mirror in front of them can also be fascinating, as babies love looking at their reflection. Getting down on the floor with your baby and engaging with them face-to-face can make tummy time more interactive and fun. Talk to your baby, sing songs, or make funny faces to keep them entertained. Your presence and interaction provide both comfort and stimulation, making tummy time a positive experience.

Sometimes, despite your best efforts, your baby might resist tummy time or seem uncomfortable. If this happens, try using a rolled blanket or a small pillow to support their chest. This slight elevation can make it easier for your baby to lift their head and look around. Encouraging brief, frequent sessions is another effective strategy. Instead of long, uninterrupted periods, break tummy time into shorter, more manageable sessions throughout the day. This approach helps build your baby's tolerance gradually without causing too much distress. Remember, it's normal for babies to fuss during tummy time initially, but with consistency and patience, they will grow more accustomed to it.

Handling tummy time challenges requires creativity and persistence. If your baby shows signs of discomfort, try different positions or use props to make them more comfortable. Sometimes, changing the environment can also help. Move to a different room or take tummy time outside on a blanket to provide a change of scenery. If your baby continues to resist, consult your pediatrician for additional tips and reassurance. They can offer guidance tailored to your baby's specific needs and help address any underlying concerns.

Incorporating tummy time into your baby's daily routine is a simple yet powerful way to support their physical development. By providing opportunities for them to strengthen their muscles and explore their surroundings, you contribute to their overall growth and well-being. Each tummy time session, no matter how brief, adds up over time, helping your baby reach important developmental milestones with confidence. Remember, the key is consistency and making the experience enjoyable for your baby. With time and practice, tummy time will become a cherished part of your daily interactions, fostering a strong foundation for your baby's future physical achievements.

Chapter 6:
Self-Care and Well-Being

I remember the first time I tried to take a moment for myself after my fourth child was born. I was standing in the shower, letting the warm water wash over me when I suddenly heard my baby crying. Instinctively, I turned off the water and rushed out, still half-soaped, to attend to her. In that moment, I realized how difficult it can be for new mothers to prioritize self-care. But I also learned that taking time for yourself isn't just a luxury—it's a necessity for your mental, emotional, and physical well-being.

Quick Self-Care Routines for Busy Moms

Self-care is essential, especially for new mothers. It can feel impossible to carve out time for yourself when you're constantly attending to your baby's needs. However, neglecting self-care can lead to burnout and decreased mental health, which impacts not only you but also your ability to care for your baby. Taking even a few minutes each day for self-care can reduce stress and improve your mood, making you a better, more patient parent.

One quick self-care practice that can make a world of difference is a five-minute meditation session. Find a quiet spot, close your eyes, and focus on your breathing. Inhale deeply through your nose, hold for a few seconds, and exhale through your mouth. This simple exercise can help center your mind and reduce anxiety. Another quick self-care activity is a stretching routine. Simple movements like neck rolls and shoulder shrugs can release tension built up from holding and feeding your baby. These exercises take only a few minutes but can leave you feeling refreshed. If you need a quick mood boost, listen to your favorite song. Music has a powerful effect on our emotions and can lift your spirits almost instantly.

Integrating self-care into your daily routine may seem challenging, but it's entirely possible with a few adjustments. For instance, turn your shower time into a mindful experience. As you wash, focus on the sensation of the water against your skin, the smell of the soap, and the sound of the water. This transforms a routine activity into a moment of relaxation. Similarly, take a moment to sip a cup of tea mindfully. Find a quiet corner, close your eyes, and savor each sip. This small break can provide a surprising amount of mental relief.

Making self-care a habit requires a bit of planning and commitment. Setting reminders on your phone can be a helpful way to ensure you take these small breaks. Schedule specific times each day for self-care activities, like a quick stretch before bed or a five-minute meditation after feeding your baby. Treat these appointments with the same importance as any other task on your to-do list. Over time, these small habits will become an integral part of your routine, providing ongoing benefits for your well-being.

Reflection Section: Creating Your Self-Care Routine
- **Morning**: Start with a five-minute meditation to set a positive tone for the day.
- **Midday**: Take a mindful shower or sip a cup of tea while your baby naps.
- **Evening**: Finish with a quick stretching routine to release the day's tension.

By integrating these quick self-care practices into your daily life, you can maintain your well-being and improve your ability to care for your baby. Remember, taking time for yourself is not selfish; it's a vital part of being a healthy, happy mother.

Restorative Yoga Poses for Postpartum Recovery

Yoga can be an excellent tool for physical and mental recovery after childbirth. It offers numerous benefits, such as increased flexibility, reduced stress, and improved circulation. For new mothers, gentle yoga is particularly suitable as it accommodates postpartum bodies still healing and adapting. Engaging in yoga helps you reconnect with your body, offering a sense of calm and stability.

Let's start with the Child's Pose. To perform this, kneel on the floor and sit back on your heels. Stretch your arms forward and lower your torso until your forehead touches the mat. This pose gently stretches the lower back, hips, and thighs, promoting relaxation. It's a restorative position that encourages blood flow and healing in the abdominal area, which can be particularly soothing after childbirth.

Next, the Cat-Cow stretch is a great way to improve spinal flexibility and posture, which often gets compromised from carrying and feeding an infant. Begin on your hands and knees in a tabletop position. Inhale as you drop your belly toward the mat, lifting your head and tailbone upward (this is the Cow Pose). Exhale and round your back toward the ceiling, tucking your chin to your chest (this is the Cat Pose). Repeat these movements, coordinating with your breath. This gentle stretch helps release tension in the spine and shoulders, offering immediate relief.

The Legs-Up-the-Wall pose is another restorative position that can be incredibly beneficial. Sit sideways against a wall and then gently swing your legs up onto the wall as you lower your back to the floor. Your body should form an L-shape. This pose helps relieve swelling and tension in the legs and feet, which can be common postpartum issues. It also encourages blood flow back to the heart and promotes relaxation.

The Reclining Bound Angle pose is perfect for opening up the hips and easing lower back discomfort. Lie on your back and bring the soles of your feet together, allowing your knees to fall open to the sides. You can use pillows or blocks under your knees for support. Rest your arms by your sides, palms facing up. This position gently stretches the inner thighs and groin, providing a sense of release and comfort.

Creating a peaceful yoga space can enhance your practice. Use a comfortable yoga mat to provide stability and cushioning. Dim lighting can create a serene atmosphere, helping you focus and relax. Playing soft, calming music can also elevate the experience, making it easier to tune into your body and breath. Consider setting up your yoga space in a quiet corner of your home where you won't be disturbed.

Consistency and Patience in Yoga Practice
Consistency and patience are essential in yoga practice. Starting with short sessions, even just ten minutes a day, can make a significant difference over time. Gradually increase the duration as you become more comfortable and confident in your practice. Accept your limitations and modify poses as needed. Your body is still healing, so it's important to listen to it. Don't push yourself too hard; the goal is to nurture your well-being, not to achieve perfection.

Yoga offers a gentle yet effective way to support your postpartum recovery. By incorporating these restorative poses into your routine, you can enjoy the physical and mental benefits they provide. Creating a calming yoga space and practicing regularly with patience and self-compassion can help you navigate the challenges of new motherhood with greater ease.

Simple Skincare Routines

As a new mother, your skin might not be your top priority, but caring for it can offer a moment of peace in your busy day. Skincare is about more than appearances; it's a form of self-care that can improve your skin's health and provide mental relaxation. Taking time for a skincare routine allows you to focus on yourself, even if only for a few minutes. This small act of self-care can make you feel more centered and rejuvenated, helping you tackle the day with renewed energy and confidence.

A quick and effective skincare routine doesn't have to be complicated. Start by cleansing your face with a gentle face wash suited to your skin type, whether dry, oily, or sensitive. A gentle cleanser removes dirt and impurities without stripping your skin of natural oils. After cleansing, use a hydrating toner to balance your skin's pH levels and provide an extra layer of moisture. This step prepares your skin to absorb subsequent products more effectively. Follow with a nourishing moisturizer to lock in hydration and keep your skin soft and supple throughout the day. Don't forget sun protection—using SPF daily is crucial to shield your skin from harmful UV rays and prevent premature aging.

Postpartum skin often faces unique challenges, such as dryness and hormonal acne. For dry skin, hydrating masks can be a lifesaver. Look for masks with ingredients like hyaluronic acid, which attracts moisture, or aloe vera, which soothes and hydrates. For hormonal breakouts, spot treatments with ingredients like salicylic acid or benzoyl peroxide can help.

Apply these treatments directly to affected areas, followed by your regular moisturizer.

Opting for natural and minimalistic skincare makes your routine more sustainable and gentle on the skin. Avoid harsh chemicals and choose products with natural ingredients such as chamomile, calendula, or green tea extract. These ingredients are effective yet less likely to irritate sensitive postpartum skin. Multi-purpose products, such as a tinted moisturizer with SPF, can simplify your routine further by combining hydration, sun protection, and light coverage in one step.

Creating a simple yet effective skincare routine can serve as a daily ritual benefiting both your skin and mental well-being. It's a small but meaningful way to reclaim some time for yourself amidst the demands of new motherhood.

Finding Time for Yourself Without Guilt

It's common for new mothers to feel an overwhelming sense of guilt when taking time for themselves. Society often pressures mothers to be constantly available and attentive to their babies, fostering the belief that any time spent away from caregiving is selfish. Internalized guilt stems from the idea that prioritizing self-care equates to neglecting your baby. This guilt can be so strong that it prevents you from doing things you enjoy or even taking a moment to rest. However, it's crucial to understand that self-care is not a luxury but a necessity for your overall well-being—and, by extension, your baby's well-being. Overcoming this guilt starts with reframing how you view self-care. Instead of seeing it as a selfish act, think of it as an investment in your health and your ability to be a better parent. Taking time for yourself helps you recharge, making you more patient and effective in caring for your baby. Setting boundaries with family members can also help manage guilt. Communicate your needs clearly and explain why taking time for yourself is important. Let them know you need their support to maintain your mental and emotional health. Open dialogue fosters understanding and respect for your need for occasional breaks.

Self-care is vital for effective parenting. When you take time to care for yourself, you increase your patience and energy, directly benefiting your baby. A well-rested and relaxed mother is better equipped to handle the challenges of caring for a newborn. Improved mental health is another benefit of self-care. By reducing stress and preventing burnout, you create a more positive and nurturing environment for your baby, helping them feel secure and loved.

Finding moments for self-care throughout the day can be challenging but is entirely possible with a bit of planning. Utilize your baby's nap times for self-care. Instead of rushing to complete chores, spend a few minutes doing something relaxing, like reading a book or taking a short walk. Enlist help from a partner or family member to carve out time for yourself. Don't hesitate to ask your partner to watch the baby for an hour while you take a bath or go for a run. Family members are often more than willing to help—they just need to know how they can support you.

Reframing your perspective on self-care, setting boundaries, and finding small moments throughout the day for yourself can significantly reduce feelings of guilt. Remember, taking time for yourself is not a sign of weakness but a step toward being the best mother you can be.

Positive Affirmations for New Moms

Positive affirmations are simple yet powerful statements that help reinforce positive thoughts and beliefs. They are particularly beneficial for new mothers, who often face a multitude of challenges and self-doubts. Positive affirmations can improve self-esteem and reduce anxiety by shifting focus from negative thoughts to empowering ones. These affirmations work by creating new neural pathways in the brain, making it easier to adopt a positive mindset over time.

For new mothers, specific affirmations can address common postpartum challenges. For instance, telling yourself, "I am doing my best, and that is enough," can be incredibly reassuring when you feel overwhelmed. This statement reminds you that perfection is not the goal—doing your best is. Another powerful affirmation is, "I am strong, capable, and resilient," which reinforces your inner strength and ability to handle the demands of motherhood. When you feel isolated or hesitant to ask for help, affirming, "It's okay to ask for help," can be liberating. It breaks down the stigma of needing assistance and encourages you to reach out. Lastly, "I am deserving of rest and self-care" is a crucial reminder that your well-being is just as important as your baby's.

Incorporating affirmations into your daily life can be straightforward and highly effective. Start by repeating affirmations in the mirror each morning. Look into your eyes and speak the words with conviction. This practice can set a positive tone for the day ahead. Writing affirmations in a journal is another excellent way to internalize them. Take a few minutes each day to jot down your affirmations, perhaps alongside your thoughts and feelings. This can serve as both a mental release and reinforcement of positive beliefs. Setting phone reminders with affirmations can also be helpful. Imagine a notification popping up in the middle of a hectic day with the message, "You are doing an amazing job." Such timely reminders can provide an instant boost.

Consistency is key when it comes to affirmations. Make them a daily habit. The more you practice, the more these positive statements will become ingrained in your mindset. Personalizing your affirmations can make them even more impactful. Create statements that resonate deeply with your specific experiences and challenges. For example, if you're struggling with breastfeeding, an affirmation like, "I am patient, and my baby and I are learning together," can be very comforting. Tailoring affirmations to your unique situation ensures they are meaningful and effective.

The power of affirmations lies in their ability to reshape thoughts and boost confidence. By consistently practicing and believing in these positive statements, you can create a more supportive and nurturing mental environment for yourself. This, in turn, allows you to face the challenges of new motherhood with greater resilience and positivity.

Mental Health Benefits of Journaling
Journaling can have a profound impact on mental well-being. Putting pen to paper allows you to process emotions, reduce stress, and increase self-awareness. When you write about your thoughts and feelings, you create an outlet for emotions that might otherwise remain bottled up. This act of expressing yourself can be incredibly therapeutic, providing a safe space to explore your inner world. You might find that simply seeing your thoughts laid out in front of you can bring clarity and a sense of relief.

Starting a journaling practice doesn't have to be daunting. Choose a journal that feels right for you, whether it's a beautifully bound notebook or a simple spiral pad. The key is to find something you're comfortable writing in. Set a regular time each day for journaling, even if it's just five or ten minutes. This consistency helps make journaling a habit, something you look forward to rather than another task on your to-do list. Early mornings or late evenings can be great times to reflect on your day and set intentions.

If you're unsure where to start, journaling prompts can help focus your writing. Consider beginning with prompts like, "What am I grateful for today?" This simple question can shift your mindset to a more positive place. Reflecting on, "What are my biggest challenges right now?" can help you identify areas where you might need support. Asking yourself, "How can I show myself kindness today?" encourages self-compassion, which is often lacking in the busy days of new motherhood. Another prompt, "What are three things I love about being a mom?" can remind you of the joys amidst the challenges. Finally, "What support do I need, and how can I ask for it?" helps you pinpoint your needs and encourages you to seek help.

Honesty and self-compassion are crucial elements of effective journaling. Write without judgment, allowing your emotions to flow freely. This is your space, and there is no right or wrong way to express yourself. Reflecting on your entries over time can also be enlightening. You'll likely notice patterns and growth that you hadn't realized before. Recognizing these changes can boost your confidence and provide a sense of accomplishment.

Remember, journaling is a tool for self-discovery and healing. It offers a moment of pause in the often chaotic world of new motherhood, giving you a chance to connect with yourself. As you continue to write, you'll find that journaling not only helps you navigate the ups and downs but also fosters a deeper understanding of your experiences and emotions. This practice can be a cornerstone of your self-care routine, providing ongoing benefits for your mental health and overall well-being.

Chapter 7:
Strengthening Relationships

The first time my husband and I tried to have a serious conversation after our fourth child was born, it was a disaster. We were both exhausted, and our tempers were short. He wanted to discuss our finances, while I just wanted a moment of peace. We ended up arguing instead of communicating. It was a wake-up call that, despite our love for each other, we needed to work on our communication skills. This chapter focuses on strengthening your relationship through effective communication, empathy, and understanding.

Effective Communication with Your Partner

Open communication is the cornerstone of any strong relationship, especially when navigating the challenges of new parenthood. Clear and honest communication helps avoid misunderstandings and fosters trust and clarity. When you and your partner can express your thoughts and feelings openly, it strengthens your emotional connection and keeps your bond strong. Without this, minor issues can escalate into significant problems, creating unnecessary stress and tension.

Practical communication strategies can make a world of difference. One effective technique is using **"I" statements** instead of **"you" statements.** For example, instead of saying, *"You never help with the baby,"* try saying, *"I feel overwhelmed when I have to handle everything on my own."* This approach focuses on your feelings without blaming your partner, making them more likely to listen without becoming defensive.

Another essential strategy is **active listening.** This means giving your full attention to your partner when they speak, maintaining eye contact, and nodding to show you understand. Reflecting back what you hear can also be helpful. For instance, if your partner says, *"I'm really stressed about work,"* you might respond, *"It sounds like work has been really tough for you lately."* This shows that you are truly listening and validating their feelings.

Scheduled check-ins can help keep communication lines open. Set aside a specific time each week to discuss any issues or concerns. This can be a quiet evening after the baby is asleep or a weekend morning over coffee. Regular check-ins ensure that both partners have an opportunity to express their feelings and address any problems before they escalate. It also creates a routine of open dialogue, making it easier to bring up sensitive topics.

Empathy and understanding play crucial roles in effective communication. Putting yourself in your partner's shoes helps you see things from their perspective. For example, if your partner is frustrated about not spending enough time with the baby, try to understand their desire to bond with your child. **Expressing gratitude** is another way to show empathy. A simple, *"Thank you for taking care of the baby last night,"* can go a long way in making your partner feel appreciated and valued. When both partners feel understood and appreciated, it strengthens their emotional connection.

Discussing sensitive topics requires careful consideration. Choosing the right time and place is essential. Avoid bringing up difficult subjects when either of you is tired or stressed. Instead, find a calm, private environment where you can talk without interruptions. Using a calm tone is equally important.

Raising your voice or using harsh words can escalate the situation. Instead, speak softly and respectfully. Collaborative problem-solving should be the goal. Work together to find solutions that satisfy both parties. For example, if you disagree about bedtime routines, discuss different options and agree on a plan that works for both of you.

Building a strong relationship through effective communication takes time and effort, but the rewards are well worth it. By using "I" statements, practicing active listening, scheduling regular check-ins, and showing empathy and understanding, you can create a foundation of trust and respect. Handling sensitive topics with care and working together to find solutions further strengthens your bond. Remember, open communication is not just about talking but also about listening and understanding each other's needs and perspectives.

Co-Parenting Strategies for New Parents

Co-parenting is an approach where both parents share the responsibilities of raising their child, regardless of their romantic relationship status. For the baby's well-being, it's crucial to ensure that both parents are actively involved, providing consistent care and support. This shared responsibility means dividing tasks equitably, from feeding and diaper changes to nighttime routines and doctor's appointments. A unified approach to child-rearing helps create a stable environment, which is essential for the baby's emotional and psychological development.

Effective co-parenting starts with creating a **solid plan.** This plan should outline each parent's roles and responsibilities clearly. For instance, you might decide that one parent is responsible for morning routines while the other handles bedtime. Regular communication is vital to keep each other updated on the baby's needs and any changes in routine.

Flexibility is also key. Babies grow and their needs change, so being able to adapt and adjust your co-parenting plan as necessary is important.

Mutual support between parents is another cornerstone of effective co-parenting. Encouraging each other with positive reinforcement can make a big difference. A simple, *"You did great with the baby last night,"* can boost your partner's confidence and strengthen your partnership. Being reliable and following through on commitments is equally important. When your partner knows they can count on you, it builds trust and reduces stress for both of you.

Disagreements are inevitable, but handling them constructively is crucial for successful co-parenting. Keeping discussions focused on the child's needs helps avoid personal attacks and keeps the conversation productive. **Seeking compromise** is essential. Finding middle ground where both parents feel heard and respected can prevent conflicts from escalating. Avoiding negative talk, especially in front of the baby, is also important. Criticizing each other can create a tense atmosphere that the baby will pick up on, even if they don't understand the words. When you co-parent effectively, you create a nurturing environment that benefits everyone involved. The baby feels secure and loved, and both parents feel supported and involved in their child's upbringing. It's a collaborative effort that requires commitment, communication, and a willingness to adapt to new challenges as they arise.

Maintaining Intimacy After Baby
The arrival of a new baby brings immense joy but can

significantly impact physical and emotional intimacy between partners. Postpartum recovery often involves physical challenges like soreness, fatigue, and hormonal fluctuations. These changes can affect your inclination toward intimacy. Sleepless nights and the constant demands of a newborn further deplete your energy for physical closeness. Additionally, the emotional shifts that come with new roles and increased responsibilities can create distance. You might find yourself so absorbed in caring for your baby that your emotional connection with your partner unintentionally takes a back seat.

To rekindle intimacy, consider scheduling date nights to prioritize couple time. Days can blur together, so planning specific moments for just the two of you can help maintain your bond. These dates don't need to be extravagant; even a simple dinner at home after the baby is asleep can be meaningful. Physical affection doesn't always need to be sexual. Holding hands, cuddling on the couch, or giving each other massages can help preserve a sense of closeness. Open communication about your desires and concerns is crucial. Discussing your feelings openly enables both partners to understand each other's needs and find ways to reconnect.

Patience and understanding are essential as you both adjust to your new roles. Accept that intimacy may evolve and look different now. It might not be the same as it was pre-baby, and that's okay. Be kind to yourself and your partner. Self-compassion and mutual support can ease the transition. Recognize that rebuilding intimacy takes time and effort from both sides. You're navigating uncharted territory together, and finding your rhythm may take a while.

Balancing baby care and couple time is challenging but

achievable with planning. Sharing baby duties is a practical approach. Alternating night shifts ensures both parents get rest and have energy for each other. This shared responsibility lightens the load and fosters mutual appreciation. Utilizing support networks also makes a difference. Enlist family or friends for babysitting, allowing you and your partner some alone time. Even a couple of hours can provide a much-needed break and an opportunity to reconnect.

Intimacy after having a baby requires conscious effort from both partners. The postpartum period is filled with new challenges and adjustments but also offers opportunities to grow closer in new ways. By scheduling date nights, maintaining physical affection, and communicating openly, you can keep your connection strong. Remember to be patient and understanding as you navigate this new phase of your relationship. Balancing baby care and couple time may involve some trial and error, but shared responsibilities and support from your network can create a nurturing environment for both your relationship and your new family.

Conflict Resolution Tips

Conflicts are inevitable in any relationship, especially during the stressful times that come with welcoming a new baby. Differing parenting styles can quickly lead to disagreements. For example, one of you might believe in a strict feeding schedule, while the other prefers a more flexible approach. Fatigue is another common source of conflict. When both partners are running on little sleep, minor issues can escalate into major arguments. Resolving these conflicts constructively is crucial for maintaining a healthy relationship. Addressing issues helps both partners feel heard and valued, strengthening the bond and fostering a harmonious home environment.

Practical conflict resolution techniques can make a significant difference. Staying calm is the first step. If your temper rises, take a break. Step away for a few minutes to collect your thoughts and return to the conversation when both of you are calmer. Using "we" statements fosters a team mindset. Instead of saying, "You never help with the baby," try, "We need to find a better way to share baby duties." This approach emphasizes collaboration rather than blame, making it easier to work together toward a solution. Finding common ground is another effective strategy. Focus on shared goals, such as wanting the best for your baby, and use that as a foundation for resolving differences.

Compromise plays a crucial role in conflict resolution. It involves negotiating and balancing individual and shared desires. For instance, if one of you wants to spend weekends visiting family while the other prefers quiet time at home, you might alternate weekends. Making concessions shows a willingness to prioritize the relationship and family. For example, you might agree to handle nighttime feedings during the week so your partner can rest for work, while they take over on weekends to give you a break. Such compromises build trust and strengthen your partnership.

Preventing future conflicts is just as important as resolving current ones. Regular check-ins can help address issues before they escalate. Set aside time each week to discuss concerns or problems. This proactive approach prevents misunderstandings and ensures both partners stay aligned. Seeking professional help is another valuable option. Couples therapy provides a neutral space to express feelings and work through conflicts constructively. A therapist can offer tailored tools and strategies to help navigate challenges more effectively.

Remember that conflicts are a normal part of any relationship, especially during the postpartum phase. Differing parenting styles and fatigue are common sources of disagreements, but resolving them constructively is essential for maintaining a healthy relationship. Staying calm, using "we" statements, and finding common ground can help resolve disputes effectively. Compromise is key to finding mutually acceptable solutions, and making concessions shows a willingness to prioritize the relationship. Preventing future conflicts through regular check-ins and seeking professional help when needed can maintain harmony and strengthen your bond.

Sharing Responsibilities Equitably
Sharing responsibilities equitably is essential for relationship harmony and overall well-being. When one partner feels overwhelmed by household and baby duties, it can lead to burnout and resentment. A fair division of labor promotes equality, fosters mutual respect, and reinforces the sense of partnership. It ensures both partners feel valued and supported, reducing stress and creating a more balanced home environment.

To divide tasks effectively, start by listing all responsibilities, from daily chores like washing dishes to nighttime feedings. Categorize these tasks and divide them based on each partner's strengths and preferences. For instance, if one of you excels at cooking, let that person handle meal preparation while the other takes on laundry. Rotating duties ensures variety and fairness, preventing either partner from feeling stuck with the same chores and fostering appreciation for each other's efforts. Flexibility is crucial when sharing responsibilities. Circumstances change, and what worked last month might not work now. Regularly re-evaluate the division of labor and be open to adjustments based on each partner's input. If one of you starts a new job or if the baby's routine changes, be willing to adapt. Open communication about workload is key. Discuss feelings of being overwhelmed or concerns openly and honestly. Transparency helps both partners understand each other's struggles and collaborate on solutions.

Seeking help when needed is also important. Despite your best efforts, managing everything on your own can become overwhelming. Hiring a babysitter or asking family members for support can provide much-needed relief, allowing both partners to recharge and maintain balance. Remember, seeking help is not a sign of failure but a practical step toward maintaining a healthy, happy home.

Equitably sharing responsibilities involves creating a list of tasks, dividing them based on strengths, and rotating duties to ensure fairness. Flexibility and open communication allow you to adapt to changing circumstances. Seeking help when necessary provides additional support. This approach reduces burnout, fosters equality, and strengthens respect and partnership, creating a harmonious environment where both partners feel valued and supported.

Building a Village: Involving Family and Friends

Involving family and friends in your parenting journey can offer substantial benefits. A strong support network provides emotional backing, helping you feel understood and less isolated. Being surrounded by people who care about you and your baby makes it easier to navigate the challenges of new parenthood. Practical help is another significant advantage. Assistance with baby care or household tasks can free up time for rest and bonding with your baby. This support can make a world of difference in managing the demands of parenting.

Building a support network begins with identifying potential helpers. Consider which family members and friends are willing and able to assist. Clearly communicate your needs, specifying the type of help you require. Whether it's babysitting, grocery shopping, or simply listening, clear communication ensures your supporters know how to help effectively. Setting boundaries is also important. Ensure that the support you receive is helpful and not intrusive by being clear about your limits and preferences.

Maintaining relationships with friends and family requires regular updates and interactions. Share baby milestones or daily happenings via social media or group chats to keep everyone involved and foster a sense of community. Make time for social interactions, even if it's just a quick coffee date or virtual hangout. These connections provide a much-needed break and emotional support.

Expressing gratitude to those who offer help is essential. A simple thank-you note or a small token of appreciation goes a long way in showing gratitude. These gestures reinforce positive relationships and encourage continued support. Acknowledging the efforts of your support network makes them feel valued, strengthening your bond with them.

Involving family and friends in your parenting journey provides emotional and practical support, easing the challenges of new parenthood. Building a support network involves identifying helpers, communicating your needs, and setting boundaries. Regular updates and social interactions maintain a sense of community, while gratitude reinforces positive relationships. This village of support can make a meaningful difference, offering the help and encouragement you need to thrive.

Sharing Responsibilities Equitably

The importance of a fair division of labor in a relationship cannot be overstated. When responsibilities are shared equitably, it prevents one partner from feeling overwhelmed and burnt out. This balance is crucial for maintaining harmony in your relationship and ensuring both partners feel valued. Sharing tasks promotes equality, fostering a sense of mutual respect and partnership. It shows that you both are in this together, working as a team to manage the demands of parenthood and household duties.

To divide tasks equitably, start by making a comprehensive list of everything that needs to be done. This can include daily chores like washing dishes, feeding the baby, and doing laundry, as well as less frequent tasks like grocery shopping and managing bills. Categorize these tasks into manageable sections. Once you have a clear list, you can begin to divide them based on each partner's strengths and preferences. If one of you is better at cooking while the other excels at organizing, play to those strengths. This not only ensures that tasks are completed efficiently but also makes the division of labor feel more balanced and fair.

Rotating duties is another effective strategy to ensure variety and fairness. If one partner always handles nighttime feedings, it can lead to fatigue and resentment. Rotating these duties gives both partners a chance to rest and recharge. This approach not only distributes the workload but also fosters empathy, as each partner experiences different aspects of childcare and household management.

Regularly re-evaluating the division of labor is equally important. As circumstances change—such as returning to work or the baby transitioning to solid foods—it's necessary to adjust responsibilities. Being open to feedback from your

90

partner and making adjustments based on their input helps maintain balance and prevents feelings of unfairness or resentment.

Flexibility is crucial when sharing responsibilities. Life with a newborn is unpredictable, and what works one week might not work the next. Regularly check in with each other to discuss how the division of labor is going, and be willing to make changes as needed. For example, you may have initially divided tasks evenly, but if one partner is struggling more, redistributing tasks can help ensure that neither feels overwhelmed. Adaptability is key to maintaining a harmonious and supportive partnership.

Maintaining balance requires open communication about workloads and a willingness to seek help when necessary. If you find yourselves struggling, don't hesitate to hire a babysitter or ask family members for support. Even a few hours of help can provide much-needed relief, allowing you to focus on other important tasks or simply rest. Discussing your challenges openly can prevent misunderstandings and ensure that both partners feel supported and valued. Acknowledging struggles and seeking help without guilt is vital for your well-being.

Task Division Exercise
Here's a simple exercise to help keep the division of labor fair and manageable:
1. **List all tasks:** Write down every household and childcare task.
2. **Categorize tasks:** Group similar tasks together (e.g., daily chores, weekly errands).
3. **Assign based on strengths:** Divide tasks according to each partner's strengths and preferences.
4. **Rotate duties:** Set a rotation schedule for demanding

or monotonous tasks.

5. **Check in regularly:** Schedule weekly or biweekly discussions to review how the division of labor is working and make adjustments as needed.

Sharing responsibilities equitably is about more than dividing tasks. It's about creating a partnership where both partners feel valued and supported. By listing, categorizing, and dividing tasks, playing to each other's strengths, and rotating duties, you can ensure a balanced workload. Flexibility and open communication are essential for adapting to changing circumstances and maintaining harmony. Seeking help and checking in regularly can prevent feelings of overwhelm and ensure a supportive, equitable partnership.

Building a Village: Involving Family and Friends

One of the most valuable lessons I learned as a new mother was the importance of building a support network. Involving family and friends can provide immense emotional and practical benefits.

Emotional support helps you feel understood and less isolated. Sharing your experiences, fears, and joys with people who care lightens the emotional load. Just knowing someone is there to listen can make a significant difference in your mental well-being.

Practical help with baby care and household tasks can free up time for rest and bonding with your baby. Whether it's a friend bringing a meal or a family member watching the baby for an hour, these small acts of kindness add up and can make a world of difference.

Building a support network starts with identifying potential helpers. Look around and consider who in your life is willing and able to help—parents, siblings, close friends, or even neighbors. Once you've identified them, communicate your needs clearly. Be specific about the type of help you need, such as someone to watch the baby while you shower or take a nap. Clear communication ensures your helpers know exactly how they can assist.

Setting boundaries is essential. Make sure the support you receive is helpful, not intrusive. Let your helpers know your preferences and limits, so they can respect your space while offering support.

Maintaining relationships with friends and family is vital for sustaining a strong support network. Regular updates about your baby's milestones and daily life can keep everyone involved and invested. Social media can help you share photos and updates with a broader circle, but don't neglect personal interactions. Coffee dates, virtual hangouts, or quick phone calls can strengthen connections. These moments provide a sense of normalcy and remind you that you're not alone.

Expressing gratitude to those who support you is crucial. Simple gestures like thank-you notes or small tokens of appreciation can go a long way. A handwritten note or a small gift, like homemade treats or a potted plant, shows your helpers how much their support means to you. Gratitude reinforces positive relationships and encourages continued support. When people feel appreciated, they're more likely to continue offering their help, creating a cycle of giving and receiving that benefits everyone.

Involving family and friends in your parenting journey offers emotional and practical support, helping you navigate the challenges of new parenthood. Building a support network involves identifying potential helpers, communicating needs clearly, and setting boundaries. Maintaining relationships through regular updates and personal interactions fosters a sense of community. Expressing gratitude to your supporters strengthens bonds and encourages ongoing support. This "village" can make a significant difference in your parenting experience, providing the help and encouragement you need to thrive.

Chapter 8:
Practical Parenting Tips and Resources

When I first became a mother, I quickly realized that managing time was one of the biggest challenges I faced. I remember days when it felt like I was constantly racing against the clock, trying to balance baby care with my personal needs. There were moments when I simply wanted to take a shower or enjoy a warm meal, but the demands of motherhood left little room for anything else. During these times, I discovered the importance of effective time management. By learning to manage my time efficiently, I reduced stress and overwhelm, creating a more balanced and fulfilling experience for both myself and my baby.

Time Management Hacks for New Mothers
Effective time management is crucial for new mothers, as it helps balance the demands of baby care with personal needs. When you manage your time well, you can reduce stress and prevent feelings of overwhelm. This balance allows you to focus on what truly matters, ensuring you have time for yourself while still meeting your baby's needs. By organizing your day and prioritizing tasks, you can create a sense of control and stability, making the early months of motherhood more manageable and enjoyable.

One of the most effective time management strategies is creating a daily schedule. Planning your day helps you allocate specific times for activities and breaks, ensuring you can attend to both your baby's needs and your own. Start by listing the essential tasks you need to accomplish each day, such as feeding, diaper changes, and naps. Then, incorporate time for self-care activities like showering, eating, and resting. Structuring your day ensures you have dedicated time for each activity, reducing the likelihood of feeling overwhelmed.

Prioritizing tasks is another crucial aspect of time management. Focus on what is essential and let go of tasks that can wait. For instance, feeding and comforting your baby should always come first. Other tasks, like household chores, can be scheduled for later or delegated to someone else. By focusing on the most important tasks, you can ensure your time and energy are spent where they are needed most. This approach helps you stay organized and reduces the pressure of trying to do everything at once.

Batch processing is a technique that involves grouping similar tasks together, allowing you to complete them more efficiently. For example, you can designate a specific time each day to respond to emails, pay bills, or run errands. By handling similar tasks in one go, you can minimize distractions and make better use of your time. This method also helps you stay focused and reduces the mental load of constantly switching between activities.

Several tools and apps can assist with time management, helping you stay organized and on track. Digital planners like Todoist and Trello are excellent for creating to-do lists and organizing tasks. These apps allow you to set reminders, prioritize tasks, and track your progress. Time-tracking apps like Toggl and RescueTime can help you monitor how you spend your time, allowing you to identify areas where you can be more efficient. By using these tools, you can streamline your daily routine and make the most of your time.

Dealing with interruptions is an inevitable part of motherhood, but flexible scheduling can help you manage these disruptions effectively. Allow for unexpected changes in your schedule by building buffer time between tasks. This flexibility ensures you can handle interruptions without feeling stressed or rushed. Additionally, use downtime effectively by tackling quick tasks during your baby's naps. For instance, you can use this time to catch up on emails, prepare a meal, or do a quick workout. By making the most of these short breaks, you can stay productive without sacrificing time with your baby.

Reflect on your time management practices and make adjustments as needed. Each day with your baby is unique, and what works one day might not work the next. Stay flexible and open to trying new strategies until you find what works best for you and your family. Remember, effective time management is not about doing more but about doing what matters most. By focusing on your priorities and making the most of your time, you can create a more balanced and fulfilling experience for both you and your baby.

Simplifying Household Chores
Managing household chores as a new mother can feel like an uphill battle. The limited time and energy you have are often consumed by the immediate needs of your baby. It's easy to feel overwhelmed when you see a pile of laundry or a sink full of dishes, knowing your baby's demands come first. The increased demands of caring for a newborn leave little room for maintaining a spotless home. It's important to recognize that it's okay not to have everything perfect. Prioritize your well-being and your baby's needs above all. Simplifying

household chores can help you find a balance, making daily life more manageable.

One effective strategy for simplifying chores is decluttering. Reducing the number of household items can significantly simplify the cleaning process. Start by going through each room and identifying items you no longer need or use. Donate or discard these items to create a more organized and manageable space. Fewer items mean less clutter and less time spent cleaning. Decluttering not only makes your home easier to maintain but also creates a more calming environment for you and your baby.

Creating a cleaning schedule can help manage household tasks more effectively. Break tasks into daily, weekly, and monthly categories to ensure everything gets done without overwhelming you. For example, daily tasks might include washing dishes, wiping down kitchen counters, and tidying the living room. Weekly tasks could involve vacuuming, mopping, and cleaning the bathroom. Monthly tasks might include deep cleaning the fridge or washing windows. By breaking tasks into manageable chunks, you can tackle them one at a time, making the process less daunting. This approach helps you stay organized and ensures that cleaning doesn't take over your entire day.

Using efficient cleaning products and tools can save time and effort. Invest in products designed to make cleaning quicker and easier. For example, microfiber cloths are excellent for dusting and wiping surfaces because they trap dust and dirt more effectively than regular cloths. Multi-purpose cleaners simplify your routine by allowing you to clean various surfaces with one product. A handheld vacuum is a quick solution for daily crumbs and small messes. These tools can help you clean more efficiently, giving you more time to focus on your baby and yourself.

Involving family members in household chores is another way to lighten your load. Assign specific tasks to each family member, ensuring clear roles for everyone. For instance, your partner can handle tasks like taking out the trash, mowing the lawn, or doing laundry. Older children can assist with simpler tasks, such as setting the table, picking up toys, or feeding pets. Rotating chores among family members ensures fairness and variety, preventing anyone from feeling overwhelmed. Sharing responsibilities not only makes chores more manageable but also fosters a sense of teamwork and cooperation within the family.

Sometimes, outsourcing chores can be a practical solution to alleviate stress. Hiring a professional cleaning service can provide significant relief, especially during the early months of motherhood. Professional cleaners can handle deep cleaning tasks, allowing you to focus on your baby and other priorities. When considering a cleaning service, think about the frequency and cost. Some families opt for weekly or bi-weekly cleanings, while others prefer monthly deep cleans. The main advantage is the time saved, which can be invaluable. However, it's essential to weigh the cost against your budget and determine if it's a feasible option for your family.

Simplifying household chores involves a combination of decluttering, creating a cleaning schedule, using efficient products, involving family members, and possibly outsourcing tasks. By implementing these strategies, you can manage your home more effectively, reduce stress, and create a more balanced life for you and your baby.

Essential Items for Baby and Mom

Bringing a newborn home requires preparation, and having the right essentials can make all the difference. **Diapers and wipes** are your first line of defense. Choosing the right type depends on your preferences and your baby's needs. Some parents prefer cloth diapers for their eco-friendliness, while others opt for disposable ones for convenience. Whichever you choose, ensure you have plenty on hand. Wipes are another necessity—look for ones that are gentle on your baby's sensitive skin and free of harmful chemicals.

Clothing basics are equally important. Stock up on onesies, sleepers, and hats. Onesies are versatile and easy to layer, making them perfect for any season. Sleepers keep your baby warm and comfortable during naps and nighttime. Don't forget hats to protect your baby's head and keep them warm, especially in cooler weather. Having a variety of sizes is helpful, as babies grow quickly.

Feeding supplies are crucial, whether you're breastfeeding or bottle-feeding. If you're breastfeeding, a good breastfeeding pillow can provide the support you need. It helps position your baby correctly, reducing strain on your back and shoulders. Bottles are essential whether you're pumping breast milk or using formula. Look for bottles with anti-colic features to help reduce gas and fussiness. Having a few different types of nipples is also helpful, as some babies have specific preferences.

Sleep essentials can significantly impact your baby's rest. A crib with a firm mattress is a must. It provides a safe sleeping environment and supports your baby's growing body. Swaddles are another sleep essential. They mimic the snugness of the womb, helping your baby feel secure and sleep better.

Swaddles can also prevent the startle reflex, which often wakes babies.

Comfortable clothing for yourself is just as important. Nursing bras and postpartum leggings offer the comfort and support you need during recovery. Nursing bras make breastfeeding more convenient, while postpartum leggings provide gentle compression to support your healing body. Personal care items like perineal spray and nipple cream can soothe discomfort and promote healing. Perineal spray helps with postpartum soreness, while nipple cream can relieve and prevent cracked nipples from breastfeeding.

Breastfeeding supplies are essential for nursing mothers. A breast pump can be a lifesaver, allowing you to express milk and store it for later use. This can be particularly helpful if you return to work or need a break. Nursing pads are another must-have. They prevent leaks and keep you comfortable and dry. Disposable nursing pads are convenient, but reusable ones are more economical and environmentally friendly.

Embracing minimalism can help you focus on essential items and avoid clutter. Quality over quantity should be your mantra. Invest in durable, useful items that will last. Multipurpose products can save space and money. For example, a baby bathtub that doubles as a storage bin or a diaper bag that can be used as a regular tote are great options. These items serve multiple functions, reducing the need for additional purchases and keeping your home clutter-free.

Creating a baby registry is a practical way to ensure you have all the essentials. Prioritize your needs by focusing on items that are most important for your baby's care and your comfort. Research products by reading reviews and seeking recommendations from other parents. This helps you choose items that are reliable and well-regarded. Including a variety of price points accommodates different budgets, making it easier for friends and family to contribute gifts that fit their financial situation.

A comprehensive approach to preparing for your baby can make the transition smoother. Having the right essentials for both your baby and yourself ensures that you're well-equipped to handle the challenges of new parenthood. Remember, focusing on quality, multipurpose items, and creating a practical registry can help you avoid unnecessary expenses and keep your home organized.

Recommended Books and Websites for Further Reading
When I had my first child, I realized how overwhelming new parenthood could be. One thing that helped tremendously was finding reliable resources to guide me through the process. Books became my go-to for comprehensive advice, and I'd like to share some that I found invaluable.

- *The Happiest Baby on the Block* by Harvey Karp is a gem that introduces the "5 Ss" method to soothe crying babies. Techniques like swaddling and shushing made a world of difference for me.
- *What to Expect the First Year* by Heidi Murkoff is another essential read, offering a month-by-month guide that covers everything from feeding to sleep schedules. This book is like having a pediatrician on call.
- *The Fourth Trimester* by Kimberly Ann Johnson focuses specifically on the postpartum period, offering practical advice for both you and your baby. It's an excellent resource for understanding the emotional and physical changes that come with new motherhood.

Helpful websites can also provide a wealth of information:

- **KellyMom** is a fantastic resource for breastfeeding support. It offers evidence-based articles and community forums where you can ask questions and share experiences.
- **BabyCenter** is another comprehensive site that covers a wide range of parenting topics. From pregnancy to toddlerhood, it's packed with articles, tips, and interactive tools like due date calculators and growth charts.
- **The Bump** offers advice on everything from pregnancy to baby care. It also has a vibrant community where you can connect with other new mothers, ask questions, and get real-time advice.

Online courses and webinars have become invaluable for continuing education. Parenting classes cover crucial topics like sleep training, baby care, and even toddler behavior. These courses are often led by experts and provide interactive learning opportunities. Webinars by pediatricians, lactation consultants, and sleep experts allow you to learn from the best without leaving your home. Many platforms also let you ask questions live, making the experience even more personalized and beneficial.

Staying informed and flexible in your parenting approach is essential. The world of parenting advice is ever-evolving, and what works for one family might not work for another. Adapting to new information is key. For instance, new research might suggest different sleep practices or feeding schedules that could benefit your family. Being open to learning and adapting ensures you're providing the best care for your baby. Seeking diverse perspectives is equally important. Exploring different parenting philosophies can offer new insights and techniques. Whether it's attachment parenting, Montessori methods, or positive discipline, each approach has its strengths.

Reflect on how these resources can fit into your parenting journey. Books, websites, online courses, and webinars each offer unique benefits. By incorporating them into your routine, you can create a well-rounded support system. Take notes, bookmark pages, and revisit sections as needed. The goal is to build a toolkit of knowledge that empowers you to make informed decisions. With these resources at your fingertips, you'll be better equipped to handle the challenges and joys of new motherhood.

Accessing Professional Services

As a new mother, you might find that professional support can make a significant difference in your journey through the fourth trimester. Accessing professional services provides specialized knowledge and expert guidance to help you navigate the complexities of newborn care and your own recovery. Professionals like pediatricians, lactation consultants, mental health specialists, and postpartum doulas offer a wealth of experience and expertise. They provide holistic care that addresses both emotional and physical needs, ensuring you and your baby receive the best support possible. This comprehensive approach helps alleviate the stress and uncertainty that often accompany new motherhood, allowing you to focus on bonding with your baby and enjoying these precious early months.

Finding and choosing the right professionals for your needs can seem daunting, but it's essential for your peace of mind and well-being.

When selecting a pediatrician for your baby, consider factors such as their experience with newborns, approach to care, and availability for emergencies. Ask for recommendations from friends, family, or your obstetrician, and schedule a meeting to see if their philosophy aligns with yours.

For breastfeeding support, a lactation consultant can be a game-changer. They offer personalized advice and hands-on assistance to help you navigate common challenges like latching difficulties and milk supply issues. Look for certified lactation consultants through local hospitals or breastfeeding support organizations.

Postpartum depression and anxiety are common, and seeking therapy can provide the support and coping strategies you need. Look for therapists who specialize in postpartum care and have experience working with new mothers. Don't hesitate to ask about their approach to treatment and how they can help you manage your symptoms.

These professionals offer in-home support that can be incredibly beneficial during the early weeks. They assist with baby care, household tasks, and provide emotional support, helping you adjust to life with a newborn. To find a postpartum doula, seek recommendations from your healthcare provider or local parenting groups.

Support groups and peer networks play a vital role in providing shared experiences and advice. Joining a local meetup or support group connects you with other new mothers who understand what you're going through. These groups offer a sense of community and emotional support, helping you feel less isolated. Local hospitals, community centers, and libraries often host parenting groups and events. Online forums and virtual support communities provide additional opportunities for connection. Platforms like Facebook and specialized parenting websites offer forums where you can ask questions, share experiences, and receive support from a broad community of parents.

Navigating healthcare systems can be challenging, but understanding how to interact with healthcare providers and insurance companies can make the process smoother. Scheduling appointments efficiently ensures you make the most of each visit. Prepare a list of questions and concerns to discuss with your healthcare provider, and take notes during the appointment. Understanding your insurance coverage is also crucial. Familiarize yourself with what's included in your plan, such as coverage for pediatric visits, lactation consultations, and mental health services. Contact your insurance provider for any clarifications and keep a record of your communications. Advocating for yourself is essential. Communicate your needs clearly and assertively, ensuring your concerns are addressed and that you receive the care you deserve.

Having access to professional support and understanding how to navigate these resources can significantly impact your postpartum experience. From selecting the right pediatrician and lactation consultant to joining support groups and understanding your insurance, these steps help create a comprehensive support system. This network of professionals and peers provides the guidance and care needed to navigate the challenges of new motherhood, ensuring that you and your baby thrive during this crucial period.

When I became a new mother, I felt an overwhelming need for connection and support. Parenting groups became a lifeline, offering a sense of community that made me feel understood and less isolated. The emotional support these groups provide is invaluable. Sharing your experiences with other new mothers who are going through similar challenges can be incredibly comforting. You realize that you're not alone in your struggles, and this shared understanding can help alleviate feelings of loneliness and anxiety.

Finding local parenting groups might seem daunting, but there are several avenues you can explore. Community centers often host parenting classes and support groups, making them a great place to start. Check local listings or visit the centers to find out what programs they offer. Hospitals and clinics are another excellent resource. Many of them run new parent groups and breastfeeding support meetings. Inquire during your prenatal visits or check with your pediatrician. Libraries also host parenting events and meetups. These gatherings can range from storytime sessions to more structured parenting workshops. Visiting your local library and asking the staff about upcoming events can lead you to valuable resources and connections.

Online parenting communities offer another layer of support, especially for those times when leaving the house feels impossible. Facebook groups are plentiful and often specific to different parenting stages, such as newborn care or toddler tantrums. These groups provide a platform to ask questions, share advice, and connect with mothers worldwide. Reddit also hosts several communities like r/Parenting, where you can find discussions on a wide range of topics. These online forums are active and engaging, offering real-time advice and support from a diverse group of parents.

Active participation in these groups can maximize the benefits you receive. Engaging with the community by asking questions allows you to seek advice and support tailored to your specific needs. Don't hesitate to share your experiences and contribute to discussions. Your insights could be invaluable to another new mother facing similar challenges. Building connections within these groups can lead to lasting friendships and a robust support network. You might find local moms to meet up with or online friends who can offer advice and companionship during late-night feedings.

Participating in parenting groups requires a bit of vulnerability, but the rewards are well worth it. These communities offer a safe space to share your fears, ask for help, and celebrate your victories. Whether you're seeking emotional support, practical advice, or simply a sense of belonging, joining a parenting group can provide the connection and reassurance you need during this transformative time.

Conclusion

As you navigate the fourth trimester, I hope this book has provided you with practical advice and emotional encouragement. The early weeks of motherhood are a profound experience, filled with moments of joy, uncertainty, and transformation. My goal has been to offer you the simplest baby guide to help both you and your little one thrive during this critical period.

In **Chapter 1**, we explored the importance of mental health. We discussed how to recognize postpartum depression versus baby blues, practical tips for managing anxiety, mindfulness exercises, and the significance of building a support network. Remember, your mental health is as crucial as your baby's well-being.

Chapter 2 focused on physical recovery and well-being. We covered healing after a C-section, pelvic floor strengthening exercises, nutritional tips for postpartum recovery, managing pain, and safe postpartum exercises. Your physical health is the foundation that will support you as you care for your baby.

In **Chapter 3**, we delved into feeding your newborn. From breastfeeding basics and overcoming common challenges to bottle-feeding tips and estimating your baby's milk needs, this chapter aimed to demystify feeding. We also touched on pumping and storing breast milk and transitioning between breast and bottle.

Chapter 4 was all about establishing sleep routines. Creating a sleep-friendly environment, understanding sleep schedules, and exploring sleep training techniques were key topics. We also discussed how to handle sleep regressions, the pros and cons of co-sleeping, and strategies for dealing with night wakings. Sleep is vital for both you and your baby.

Chapter 5 highlighted newborn care essentials. We covered interpreting baby cues, bath time basics, diapering, handling common baby ailments, safe babywearing techniques, and the importance of tummy time. These practical tips ensure you are well-equipped to care for your baby.

In **Chapter 6**, we turned the spotlight on self-care and well-being. Quick self-care routines, restorative yoga poses, simple skincare routines, and the importance of finding time for yourself were discussed. Positive affirmations and the mental health benefits of journaling were also emphasized. Taking care of yourself is not a luxury; it's a necessity.

Chapter 7 focused on strengthening relationships. Effective communication with your partner, co-parenting strategies, maintaining intimacy, conflict resolution tips, sharing responsibilities equitably, and involving family and friends were key points. A strong support system is essential for your emotional health and your baby's well-being.

Chapter 8 provided practical parenting tips and resources. Time management hacks, simplifying household chores, essential items for both baby and mom, recommended books and websites, accessing professional services, and joining local and online parenting groups were covered. These tools and resources are designed to make your journey smoother.

The most important messages in this book are simple yet profound: Take care of your mental and physical health. Build a support network. Be patient and kind to yourself. Remember, you are not alone. Reach out for help when you need it, and celebrate the small victories along the way. Each step you take is a testament to your strength and resilience.

Proactively apply what you've learned. Set up a routine that works for you and your baby. Practice the self-care techniques that resonate with you. Communicate openly with your partner and involve them in parenting duties. Connect with other new mothers to share experiences and support each other.

As a mother of five and a naturopathic doctor, I understand the challenges and joys of the fourth trimester. You are doing an incredible job. Your baby is thriving because of your love and care. Both of you are on a path to health, happiness, and well-being.

In closing, I want to leave you with a message of hope and encouragement. You are resilient and capable. The fourth trimester is a time of monumental change, but with the right guidance and support, you can overcome any challenge. Trust in your abilities and know that you have the strength to navigate this journey successfully. You and your baby are embarking on a beautiful adventure together, and every day is a new opportunity to grow and bond.

Thank you for allowing me to be a part of your journey. I wish you and your baby all the love, joy, and health in the world.

References

10 Cleaning Tips for Busy Moms & Dads
   https://www.mollymaid.com/practically-
   spotless/2022/january/cleaning-tips-for-busy-moms/
5 Mindfulness Practices for Surviving New Parenthood
   https://medium.com/thrive-global/5-mindfulness-
   practices-for-surviving-new-parenthood-
   61cf60317547
7 expert tips on how to co-parent successfully - BabyCenter
   https://www.babycenter.com/family/parenting-
   styles/co-parenting_41001524
Amount and Schedule of Baby Formula Feedings
   https://www.healthychildren.org/english/ages-
   stages/baby/formula-feeding/pages/amount-and-
   schedule-of-formula-feedings.aspx
Baby bath basics: A parent's guide
   https://www.mayoclinic.org/healthy-lifestyle/infant-
   and-toddler-health/in-depth/healthy-baby/art-
   20044438
Breastfeeding with Sore Nipples https://llli.org/breastfeeding-
   info/breastfeeding-sore-nipples/
Breathing exercises for stress - NHS https://www.nhs.uk/mental-
   health/self-help/guides-tools-and-
   activities/breathing-exercises-for-stress/
Calming Postnatal Yoga Sequence for the 'Fourth Trimester'
   https://www.yogajournal.com/yoga-101/types-of-
   yoga/prenatal/calming-postpartum-yoga-sequence-
   for-the-fourth-trimester/
Cloth Diapers vs. Disposable Diapers: Which Should I Use?
   https://www.whattoexpect.com/diapering-
   essentials/cloth-vs-disposables.aspx
Common Infant and Newborn Problems

https://medlineplus.gov/commoninfantandnewborn
problems.html

Conflict management for parents
https://raisingchildren.net.au/grown-ups/looking-
after-yourself/communication-conflict/conflict-
management-for-parents

C-section recovery: Timeline, aftercare tips, and expectations
https://www.babycenter.com/baby/postpartum-
health/c-section-recovery_221

Explore Postpartum Depression in the United States | AHR
https://www.americashealthrankings.org/explore/me
asures/postpartum_depression

Ferber Method for Sleep Training: A Parent's Guide - Babies
https://www.parents.com/baby/sleep/basics/the-
ferber-method-explained/

Getting a good latch | Office on Women's Health
https://www.womenshealth.gov/breastfeeding/learni
ng-breastfeed/getting-good-latch

Have a Baby and Still Want to Get Things Done?
https://www.nytimes.com/article/new-parents-time-
management-guide.html

How to communicate with your partner after having a baby - NCT
https://www.nct.org.uk/life-parent/your-
relationship-couple/relationship-challenges-and-
support/how-communicate-your-partner-after-
having-baby#:~:text=Remember%20to%20listen,-
Communication%20is%20a&text=It's%20difficult%2
0sometimes%20but%20try,listen%20to%20you%20b
etter%20too%20.

Kegel exercises: A how-to guide for women
https://www.mayoclinic.org/healthy-
lifestyle/womens-health/in-depth/kegel-
exercises/art-20045283

Learning your baby's cues https://www.marchofdimes.org/find-
support/topics/neonatal-intensive-care-unit-
nicu/learning-your-babys-cues

Must Read Parenting Books for New Parents

https://www.alifewellconsumed.com/must-read-
parenting-books-for-new-parents/

Newborn Baby Checklist—The Must-Haves and More
https://www.pampers.com/en-
us/pregnancy/preparing-for-your-new-
baby/article/newborn-baby-checklist

Nurturing Intimacy: A Guide to Sex and Connection After ...
https://www.postpartum.net/nurturing-intimacy-a-
guide-to-sex-and-connection-after-childbirth/

Paced Bottle-Feeding: How to Mimic Breast-Feeding
https://www.healthline.com/health/parenting/paced
-bottle-feeding

Postpartum care: After a vaginal delivery
https://www.mayoclinic.org/healthy-lifestyle/labor-
and-delivery/in-depth/postpartum-care/art-20047233

Postpartum depression - Symptoms and causes
https://www.mayoclinic.org/diseases-
conditions/postpartum-depression/symptoms-
causes/syc-20376617

Postpartum Nutrition Tips to Help Support Recovery
https://www.nutritionnews.abbott/pregnancy-
childhood/prenatal-breastfeeding/postpartum-
nutrition-tips-to-help-support-recovery/

Skincare guide for new moms: 8 dermatologist-approved ...
https://www.hindustantimes.com/lifestyle/health/sk
incare-guide-for-new-moms-8-dermatologist-
approved-tips-for-achieving-postpartum-glow-
101715594987030.html

Supportive Benefits of Journaling for Postpartum Mental ...
https://wellmindperinatal.com/358-supportive-
benefits-of-journaling-for-postpartum-mental-health/

The Best Types of Blackout Curtains for Better Baby Sleep
https://sleepoutcurtains.com/blogs/home/the-best-
types-of-blackout-curtains-for-better-baby-sleep-a-
comprehensive-guide?srsltid=AfmBOoqISi52z-
Lv3Ge2bgZZTXNb87NqoW2TC3BnCt8_juK_Tiim
Wss3

The Best White Noise Machine
    https://www.nytimes.com/wirecutter/reviews/best-white-noise-machine/
This Is Self-Care: 10 Tips for New Moms
    https://www.kindredbravely.com/blogs/bravely/self-care-tips-new-moms
What Is the Best Room Temperature for Baby?
    https://www.healthline.com/health/baby/room-temperature-for-baby

www.ingramcontent.com/pod-product-compliance
Lightning Source LLC
Chambersburg PA
CBHW071015120626
46546CB00003B/1104